#1350

WEIGHT LOSS SURGERY

A LIGHTER LOOK

...AT A HEAVY SUBJECT

WRITTEN BY
TERRY SIMPSON, MD, FACS

Terry Simpson
5-17-04

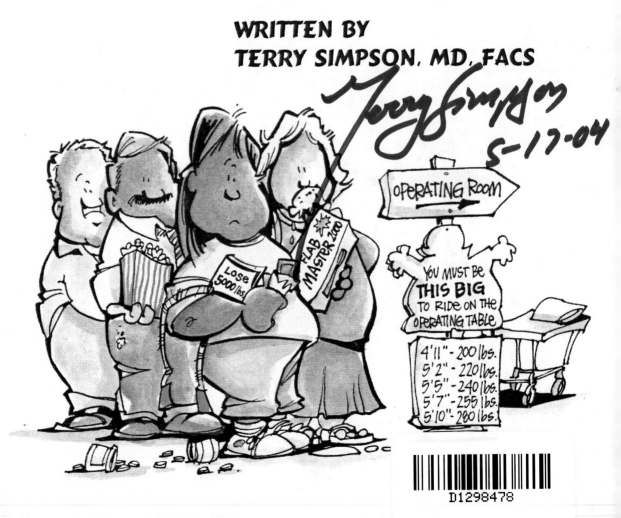

OPERATING ROOM

YOU MUST BE **THIS BIG** TO RIDE ON THE OPERATING TABLE

4'11" - 200 lbs.
5'2" - 220 lbs.
5'5" - 240 lbs.
5'7" - 255 lbs.
5'10" - 280 lbs.

D1298478

© Copyright 2004 Terry Simpson. All rights reserved.

No part of this publication may be reproduced, stored in a retrieval system, or transmitted, in any form or by any means, electronic, mechanical, photocopying, recording, or otherwise, without the written prior permission of the author.

Printed in Victoria, Canada

Note for Librarians: a cataloguing record for this book that includes Dewey Classification and US Library of Congress numbers is available from the National Library of Canada. The complete cataloguing record can be obtained from the National Library's online database at: www.nlc-bnc.ca/amicus/index-e.html

ISBN 1-4120-2283-5

TRAFFORD

This book was published on-demand in cooperation with Trafford Publishing. On-demand publishing is a unique process and service of making a book available for retail sale to the public taking advantage of on-demand manufacturing and Internet marketing. On-demand publishing includes promotions, retail sales, manufacturing, order fulfilment, accounting and collecting royalties on behalf of the author.

Suite 6E, 2333 Government St., Victoria, B.C. V8T 4P4, CANADA

Phone   250-383-6864   Toll-free   1-888-232-4444 (Canada & US)
Fax   250-383-6804   E-mail   sales@trafford.com

Web site www.trafford.com TRAFFORD PUBLISHING IS A DIVISION OF TRAFFORD HOLDINGS LTD.

Trafford Catalogue #04-0111   www.trafford.com/robots/04-0111.html

10   9   8   7   6   5   4   3

Thanks

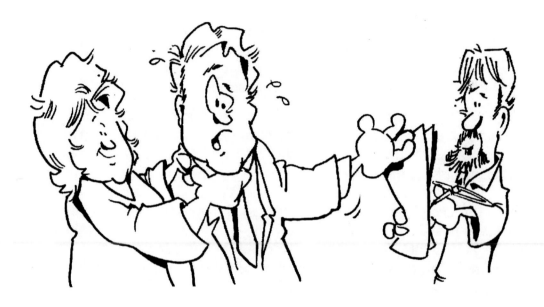

I could not have completed this book without the help of my editor, Yvonne Gray, and my illustrator, Jim Hunt. My editor had infinite patience (as you can see) and somehow my illustrator just keeps drawing away. Thanks, Von, for not shooting the author.

Dedication

I dedicate this book to my patients and friends from the Gila River Indian Reservation.

The year that I finished my surgical residency, I went to work for the Indian Health Service in Phoenix where I was assigned to a clinic on the Gila River Indian Reservation. I have continued to maintain a clinic at Hu Hu Kam Memorial Hospital, the hospital that serves the reservation, since 1991.

From the beginning, I felt a kinship with my patients. That is probably because these first patients are my distant cousins. I am of Athabascan heritage (interior Alaska Native). These were the first "snowbirds," migrating from our home in Alaska to the Southwest thousands of years ago where for many years they lived a peaceful existence along the banks of the Gila River. Then the white man came and formed reservations. They also brought with them white bread, white sugar, and lots of lard. As a result, this small reservation has the highest incidence of adult-onset diabetes and morbid obesity of any group of people in the world. Their cousins, who live in Northern Mexico, do not enjoy this bounty of dense, fat-laden carbohydrates and do not have problems with obesity or diabetes.

I have learned a lot from these patients. I learned to laugh, and I learned that if you feel "no way," that is a good thing—but if you feel "some way," then something is wrong. So, for Troy, Tony, Robert, Patricia, and a thousand other patients who have taught me so much—thank you. Just remember—drink a lot of water. It may be only 117 degrees outside, but it is a dry heat!

Also dedicated to...

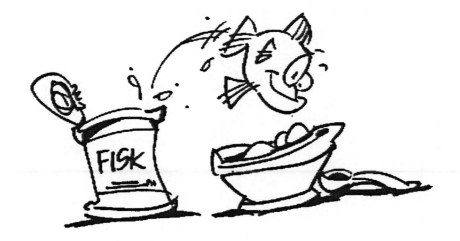

Contents

Part 1

Pre-Op

Part 2

Surgery

Part 3

Early Post-Op

Part 4

Recipes & Meal Plans

Part 5

Appendices

Appendix Three

Appendix Four

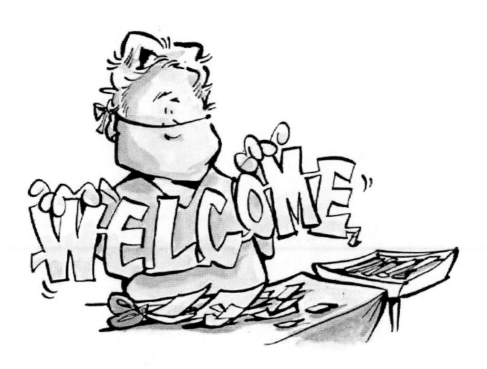

Part 1

Pre-Op

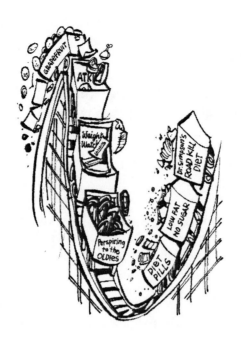

One

Diet and Exercise

There are alternatives to weight loss surgery. Diet and exercise do work but, instead of developing a new routine and new habits, patients fall back to old habits and regain their lost weight (it never really is lost, is it?). In fact, you cannot dispute that diet and exercise are critical to the success of weight loss surgery. You can go a step further and say that if you follow a reasonable routine of diet and exercise like the ones outlined in this book, you will not need any form of surgery.

The laughing you hear in the background is from my friends who have gone through this before. Okay gang! Quiet down. We might have some righteous skinny person reading this book telling their vertically-challenged friend, "See, Dr. Simpson agrees—you just need to... blah, blah, blah."

The reason we surgeons do weight loss surgery is because there is a point where patients get tired of the cycle—or recidivism. That's a great word. It means falling back to old habits. The National Institute of Health reports that

95 percent of people who are morbidly obese will regain lost weight within two years.

Ah oh, here come those righteous preachers again—they are going to tell you all about willpower. Let me just list those lines in this book for those who don't wish to contemplate weight loss surgery and want to think about diet and exercise:

(1) You just need to…

(2) You just need more willpower.

(3) Try this pill (pick one). God knows what is in some of these pills you can buy without a prescription, and doesn't it make you feel good to know that there are no government regulations about these pills or their claims of being safe and effective?

(4) Do this workout (pick your favorite skinny star who is pawning a tape or DVD of their plastic surgery-reconstructed body doing some workout).

(5) Try this machine. Oh, the infomercials—you have to love these. There are machines that make you feel like it really isn't exercise! There are machines that are "designed" to make you lose weight in 30, 45, or 90 days. I have owned a couple of machines and found that they make a great place to hang clothes.

(6) Lose weight while you sleep (for those who slept through the class where you learned about PT Barnum and a sucker born every minute).

(7) Biofeedback (as if food isn't the world's greatest biofeedback).

(8) Behavior modification (just strap these electrodes on your…).

(9) Try this prescription (to see last year's favorite weight loss drug, check the yellow pages under legal firms). Of course, some weight loss drugs work well. Amphetamines and cocaine are two great examples—but they will kill you faster than obesity.

A multibillion-dollar industry is built around obesity. There is everything from fad diets that make you pass gas or eat roadkill, to pills that contain stimulants like ephedrine that can, and do, kill people. There is a diet for every food group—the protein diet, the carbohydrate diet, the fat diet, the sugar diet. There is a diet for every food. There is the rice diet, the grapefruit diet, the salami diet, the cabbage soup diet. There are diets that are low in carbohydrates, and diets that are low in protein. Fat is good. No, it is bad.

Confused yet? Even the world's "experts," cannot agree. I loved seeing the late Dr. Atkins and Dr. Ornish go at each other; it was more fun than watching wrestling. There is more arguing about the "best" diet than there is arguing about whose church to worship in. Then there are those who say that the answer is not food, it is vitamins and supplements—but not just any vitamin or supplement, you must have the one they are selling (what a shock). Why eat, just take these pills with this powder, mix it with this bottled water or skim milk (blue water) and you are on your way to weight loss. Soyant green is the best for this (for later generations see The Matrix, and what that machine feeds its batteries).

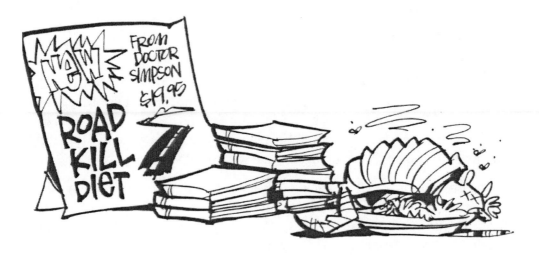

Even doctors disagree and we have degrees in medical science. There is both legitimate science here and a lot of whooie. So how do you sort the pearls from the swine??? That brings me to my favorite myths from "nutrition stores." You will hear people say, "Doctors really don't have any training in nutrition." This is, by the way, completely wrong and misleading. How do they know? (Oh, I forgot. They went to medical school but gave up medicine to peddle vitamins in the strip mall and are now experts about nutrition.) Some claim they formulate their product just for you. Can you hear it now? President of XYZ Vitamin Company is saying, "You know, Dr. Simpson is putting on a few pounds. Let's formulate something for a five-foot nine-inch, tall, handsome male doctor."

Why do you need a doctor? There is an army of self-proclaimed experts willing to give you advice. Sometimes it is free but most of the time it costs something. Sometimes it is your skinny sister-in-law whose idea of weight-gain is the five pounds she gained during her fifth pregnancy. Those are the easy ones to dismiss. The harder ones are those who have the answer for just a few dollars a month. "Sad, tired all the time, feel lonely? Join our cult."

Obese patients are prey for every device, food supplement, motivational speaker, vitamin, and diet. Everyone has advice, everyone has an answer. You need religion, your problem is religion, you need more self-esteem, you have too much self-esteem, you need therapy, and you don't need therapy. Join this group, join this gym, and call my trainer. Jog. No, walk. No, run—run marathons.

Diets work. You can always lose weight on diets, but keeping the weight off is the issue.

Then there is the ethnic diet-of-the-year club. The Himalayans: "They eat this weird yogurt that only we sell." Or the Norwegians— "These people live longer because they eat cod soaked in lye." Funny, no one has ever recommended that we go on an English diet. Then again, maybe that should be my next book. Who wouldn't lose weight eating English cooking? It is definitely one way to eat smaller portions.

The great thing about ethnic diets is that you can select almost any country, people, or race in the world and point out how skinny they are. Except Americans. Try this experiment: go to almost any foreign country, and if you find an overweight couple walking down the street ask where they are from. More than likely, they will say they are from the United States.

Diets work. You can always lose weight on diets, but keeping the weight off is the hard part. Most weight loss surgeons require their patients to lose weight before surgery. This may not make sense to you, but it makes perfectly good sense to the doctor. First, after surgery patients will not regain the weight they lost. Second, it shows a commitment to follow through after surgery. The issue for all of weight loss surgery is the aftercare. Weight loss surgery is not a quick fix; it is a marker for a change in lifestyle. Weight loss surgery is not for those who plan to have the surgery and then resume their prior lifestyle. It doesn't work that way.

Here is a simple quiz. Diets don't work because:

(a) you cannot eat cabbage soup forever.

(b) you have a stomach capable of digesting large mammals and you want it filled with one.

(c) your intestines are so absorbent that Phoenix air (which has little oxygen and lots of calories) causes you to gain weight.

(d) all of the above.

Celebrities have the answer to staying thin. Of course, they also have personal trainers, personal chefs, and vitamin companies putting them on retainer to promote their products. My favorite celebrities are the ones who rail against weight loss surgery, then bring to their show patients who have had weight loss surgery that failed to keep them thin and healthy. These people don't have the answer for sustained weight loss for everyone, or ironically, even for themselves. My patients are not celebrities. My patients are like Scott, a single dad with three boys and two jobs who wants to be around to play with his grandkids. He can't afford to join a gym and doesn't have the time.

So, if you are morbidly obese or know someone who is, this book is for you. We will tell you all about weight loss surgery—the good, the bad, and the ugly. We will also tell you about after-care. More than with any other surgery, the after-care programs for weight loss surgery patients are critical.

Weight loss surgery is unlike any other surgery. That is why there are lots of support groups for patients. Appendectomy patients or patients who have had their gallbladder removed don't need support groups.

There are so many myths about weight loss surgery that I felt it was time to eliminate the confusion and explain the program in this book.

Why Do We Get Fat?

—or, are your genes making you wear larger jeans?

The Pima Indians in Southwest Arizona have one of the highest rates of diabetes in the nation. Diabetes and obesity were unknown to these Indians prior to the coming of the white man and his white bread. Their cousins who live in Northern Mexico have the same genetic background but they don't have the rich diet that Americans have, therefore they don't have a problem with obesity.

Those of you who are nature versus nurture-types might think—ah ha, the problem is clearly environmental, but it is not. The predisposition of Pima Indians toward obesity is genetic. Add that to a diet filled with lots of sugar and fat, and you have obesity.

The teleological reason for this is in what we call the "feast or fast gene." The reasoning goes like this—while Arizona is a great place to have a winter vacation, it is a desert. Thousands of years ago people had to scrape out a living in the desert. Famine was not uncommon. Those who were blessed with a feast/fast gene had the ability to store great quantities of food (as fat) in times of plenty. When the famine struck, those little skinny guys didn't make it, but those with the feast/fast gene did. Generations later, the children of those who survived have bodies that are particularly well suited to storing fat during good times and surviving during the famine. Now I have a secret to tell those survivalists who have basements full of canned goods. Being fat is the best protection against famine. Someone can steal the food out of your basement, but if you store your reserves as fat—well, then again there was the Donner Pass Party.

Then we entered the era of modern transportation, fast food, and television. No more famines, at least not in the United States. So, now some people simply store, and store, and store. These are the ones who become obese.

What is the best remedy? More famines? Well, some government bureaucrat might think so, but it probably won't become policy. Leaders in the Zuni Nation came up with one of the best remedies I have heard of. They took a group of young school kids and started them on a program of running and exercise. What a wonderful model. Remember, exercise is the great equalizer—and this program will instill healthy values in children that will pay dividends later.

Now the academic people will point to some interesting research with various proteins, other genetic studies, and hold a long and boring discussion about obesity. But suffice it to say, there is clearly a genetic predisposition to obesity. This predisposition is boosted by our modern sedentary lifestyle, which has a bountiful supply of calories in concentrated and delicious forms.

The ultimate question is this: will modern science someday find a pill or shot or something that will decrease that trend? I hope so, but probably not in our lifetime. I would love to save patients the scar and hand them a pill. Meanwhile, read this book.

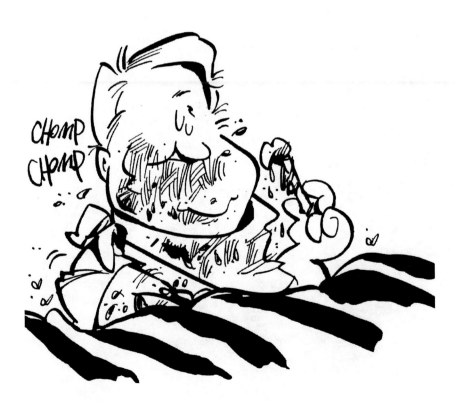

Not a Disclaimer

I am a physician, but I am not *your* physician. While my advice in this book is simple, easy to follow, and is based on years of experience as a weight loss surgeon, it cannot take the place of your doctor, the one who sees you, examines you and knows your insides. The same is true for physicians, friends, and other health care workers who you meet in restaurants, bars, and the internet or on the street. Trust your doctor. If he disagrees with me—well, go with his recommendations. You are paying for his advice about you. You can get a second opinion if you don't trust your doctor's advice. In fact, if you don't trust your doctor's advice, maybe you should get another doctor. If you are my patient, then trust what I say in here as absolute gospel and have this book burned on the fleshy tables of your heart.

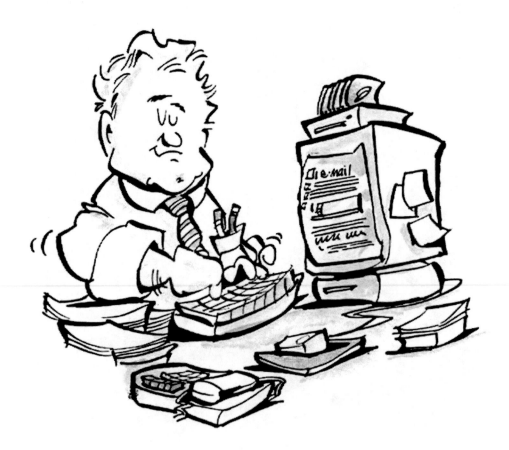

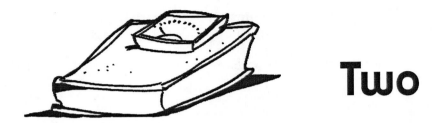

What Is Morbid Obesity?

So, what is morbid obesity, and why do we care? I could bore you with Greek or Latin derivatives—such as, "morbid" means death and "obesity" means fat, and you might conclude that morbid obesity means death fat. That is a cute interpretation but also accurate. I can even assign figures to morbid obesity—or I can tell you what a Supreme Court member said about pornography and apply it to morbid obesity: "I know it when I see it."

We all know the upper end of morbid obesity when we see it. A 500-pound person is hard not to notice. However, not many of my patients weigh 500 pounds. Most are between 200 and 300 pounds. One question my patients ask is, just how morbidly obese do they have to be to have surgery? We have a way of calculating your height-to-weight ratio called the body mass index. If your height and weight reach a certain level, then you are eligible for weight loss surgery. If your body mass index is over 40, you are eligible for surgery. If it is over 35 and you have certain "co-morbidities," you are eligible for surgery.

How We Measure Obesity

—finally, Dr. Simpson, give us something

Both the National Institute of Health (NIH) and the World Health Organization (WHO) endorse BMI (Body Mass Index) as the measurement of obesity.

The formula is: BMI = weight in kg / height in meters X height in meters.

Underweight	BMI < 18.5 kg/m²
Normal Range	BMI 18.5-24.9 kg/m²
Overweight	BMI 25- 30 kg/m²
Class I obesity	BMI 30- 34.9 kg/m²
Class II obesity (aka morbid obesity)	BMI 35 – 39.9 kg/m²
Class III obesity	BMI 40 -49.9 kg/m²
Class IV obesity	BMI > 50 kg/m²

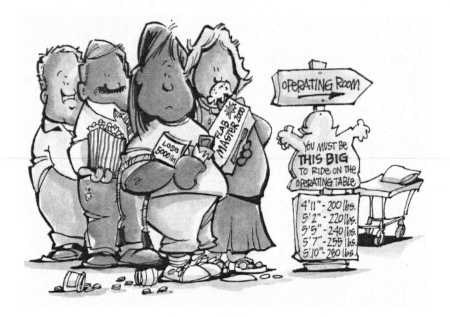

BMI Chart

The following table list the major BMIs. Find your height and then locate your weight in the same row. If your weight is below the BMI of 35, then you are not eligible for most weight loss surgery. If your BMI is more than 40, then you are eligible for weight loss surgery. See Appendix One, page 5-13, for BMIs of 25 to 50.

Height in inches	BMI of 35	BMI of 40	BMI of 45	BMI of 50
4'10"	167 lbs	191 lbs	215 lbs	239 lbs
4' 11"	174 lbs	198 lbs	233 lbs	248 lbs
5' 0"	179 lbs	205 lbs	230 lbs	256 lbs
5' 1"	185 lbs	212 lbs	238 lbs	265 lbs
5' 2"	191 lbs	219 lbs	246 lbs	273 lbs
5' 3"	198 lbs	226 lbs	254 lbs	282 lbs
5' 4"	204 lbs	233 lbs	262 lbs	291 lbs
5' 5"	211 lbs	241 lbs	271 lbs	301 lbs
5' 6"	217 lbs	248 lbs	279 lbs	310 lbs
5' 7"	224 lbs	256 lbs	288 lbs	320 lbs
5' 8"	230 lbs	263 lbs	296 lbs	329 lbs
5' 9"	237 lbs	271 lbs	305 lbs	338 lbs
5' 10"	244 lbs	279 lbs	313 lbs	348 lbs
5' 11"	251 lbs	287 lbs	322 lbs	358 lbs
6' 0"	259 lbs	295 lbs	332 lbs	369 lbs
6' 1"	265 lbs	303 lbs	341 lbs	379 lbs
6' 2"	272 lbs	311 lbs	350 lbs	389 lbs
6' 3"	280 lbs	320 lbs	360 lbs	400 lbs
6' 4"	288 lbs	329 lbs	370 lbs	411 lbs

Fat Rats

Class IV obesity has been added to the Morbid Obesity list by many bariatric surgeons, as people with this class have increased risks from their obesity. Some studies show that a BMI of greater than 60 kg/m^2 represents a special class of "Super Morbid Obesity" and has greater surgical and other risks.

If you get the hint that the "morbid" part of morbid obesity means that fat is more than just a cosmetic problem, you are correct. People are not like ice cream— ice cream tastes better with a high fat content, the same with steaks— we like a well-marbled meat. People do not do well with a higher fat content, although I have not checked with my local cannibal friends. There are lots of diseases associated with increased weight, so there are lots of reasons to lose that weight. It's also probable that if you fit into the obese category, you will only lose weight, and keep it off, with surgery.

Section Three of this book is about diets. This chapter, however, is just to help you understand why carrying around a few extra pounds might not be the best thing for you.

You just are not going to find a lot of old folks who could stand to lose 80 pounds or more—old is a relative term. I suspect we all feel that "old" is anyone ten years older than we are, but let us define old as 85 years or greater. Many scientific studies show rats live longer when their calories are limited. I live in a citrus grove in Arizona, and when "roof rats" started to overrun the neighborhood, the city officials wanted to pick all the citrus and starve them. I said, "Let the little buggers gorge themselves. It will be much easier for the cats to get them."

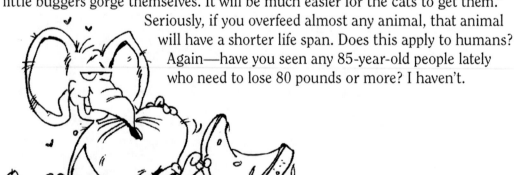
Seriously, if you overfeed almost any animal, that animal will have a shorter life span. Does this apply to humans? Again—have you seen any 85-year-old people lately who need to lose 80 pounds or more? I haven't.

Which is Worse, Cigarettes or Obesity?

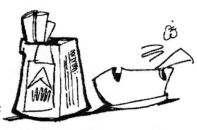

Many other things that are bad for you don't necessarily shorten your life span. Your average smoker, while puffing away on his second pack, will tell you how Aunt Mabel lived to be 100 years old even though she smoked a couple packs a day. You will also hear how Uncle George drank a fifth of scotch after drinking a case of beer and died in his 90's. Then there are those aging rock stars who continue to support heroine habits and party heartily while still going on tour. But guess what? None were overweight—at least not enough to fit into the morbid class. It is easy to find someone who managed to escape the ravages of obvious tobacco, alcohol, or drug abuse, or who lived in a toxic waste dump, and yet no family members, other than their two-headed turtle, suffered ill effects. But obesity is another matter. The body isn't built for that kind of abuse. So, in terms of lengthening your life, one of the best things you can do for yourself is to be thin. On the other hand, if you want to live a short life—gain 80 pounds. Maybe I should send my mother-in-law some more chocolates?

Why is morbid obesity such a problem? Wow, what a great question. The answer is that almost every organ, every muscle in your body, can become invested with fat, and a lot of diseases are associated with this extra fat. Here is a list of some of those diseases and their relationship to obesity.

Obesity-related disease that can limit your life

- heart disease
- Type II Diabetes
- high blood pressure
- cancer
- fatty liver disease
- sleep apnea (narcolepsy)
- elevated blood levels of cholesterol and/or lipids

Co-morbidities

–those mentioned by the NIH

In certain instances, less severely obese patients (with BMIs between 35 and 40) also may be considered for surgery. Included in this category are patients with high-risk co-morbid conditions such as life-threatening cardiopulmonary problems (e.g., severe sleep apnea, Pickwickian syndrome, and obesity-related cardiomyopathy) or severe diabetes mellitus. Other possible indications for patients with BMIs between 35 and 40 include obesity-induced physical problems interfering with lifestyle (e.g., joint disease treatable but for the obesity, body size problems precluding or severely interfering with employment, family function, and ambulation).

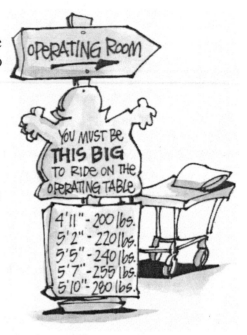

Heart Disease

Heart disease has long been associated with obesity. It's not hard to figure out why. The diet of obese patients has all the ingredients to coat the arteries with plaque (artery-clogging plaque, not the kind you get on your teeth). Pumping against a hundred extra pounds will soon take a toll on the heart.

What is plaque? Plaque is atherosclerosis, or arteriosclerosis (fun with words again—it roughly translates to "hard porridge," which is what these plaques are like—that skimmy stuff on top and that soft stuff in the middle). Plaque is a substance that coats the artery and narrows it. If the artery becomes narrowed enough then not enough blood can get to the tissues or an organ.

As the build-up of atherosclerosis occurs in the arteries going to the heart muscle, less and less blood gets to that muscle. Sometimes the muscle develops a specific pain, which we call "angina." If one of those patches of plaque blocks the artery completely, then the heart muscle will eventually die and you will have a heart attack (or, a "coronary" as some folks call it, because the coronary artery is blocked). If the heart muscle isn't receiving enough blood to do its job, then the heart won't work well and problems, such as congestive heart failure, will develop.

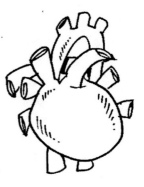

Some of the plaque buildup is due a high cholesterol level. A certain percent of blood cholesterol comes from what you eat. Doctors debate over which foods cause a rise in that cholesterol: some argue it is caused by eating too many carbohydrates, others that it is caused by a diet rich in fats. That issue will be debated for a long time. No matter which doctor's theory you might believe, obese people have diets that contain plenty of foods that build plaque in the arteries. There is some good news. Some drugs greatly decrease cholesterol and lipids in the blood, but they are rather expensive. The best news is that research has shown if you lose weight and decrease the amount that you eat (both of which happen with surgery), this buildup of plaque will reverse itself a bit. So, here is yet another reason to turn down that second plate.

Heart disease is the most common reason people die in the United States, and it is clearly related to diet and obesity. Weight loss surgery allows a person to decrease the risk of heart disease from obesity, and if patients change their diet because of the surgery, they eliminate yet another risk factor of heart disease. Another way is to eat fish—the fat in fish actually protects you from heart disease a bit. Fish is a great source of protein, a good source of the types of fats that are protective, and if you get them fresh, they are downright tasty. Try Halibut with Macadamia nut topping—mmmm.

Diabetes Mellitus

There is a recent rise in the incidence of adult onset diabetes, or Diabetes Mellitus (DM) Type II, and this rise is directly related to obesity. Diabetes has two forms, Type I and Type II. Type II Diabetes is an inability to use the insulin properly. Simply put, the more fat cells you have, the more insulin you will require. Think of fat cells as a huge sponge that soaks up insulin. Type I Diabetes, also called juvenile diabetes, is caused from a lack of production of insulin by the pancreas. This occurs mostly in children, although it also sometimes occurs in young adults.

Weight loss will increase the body's ability to use its own insulin. So, if you have Type I Diabetes and lose weight, you will probably not require as much insulin as you did before. If you have Type II DM, you may also require less insulin, fewer pills, or you may even be able to get off the medication for DM entirely. Insulin helps the body convert blood sugar into useful fuel. If you have a high blood sugar level, that means you are not using it as fuel and this can lead to diabetes and a host of problems that come with it. Diabetes is directly linked to heart disease, obesity, blindness, strokes, and loss of legs. If you have DM and are treated for it, you will have more energy, be able to do more of the things that you enjoy doing, and feel much better overall.

High blood sugar levels will also make you quite thirsty as well as make you urinate more. I am a bit of a hypochondriac. Okay, being a doctor means that I am more than a bit. I don't get headaches, I get brain tumors—undiagnosed and untreated they go away. One weekend, during a hot Arizona summer, I was golfing with my friends. It was 105-110 degrees so I drank a lot of water, along with iced tea, in the clubhouse. I worked with Pima Indians who have the highest incidence of Type II Diabetes in the world, and have the same genetic background as I do (I am one quarter Alaska Native—Athabascan to be exact), and I was convinced I was going to get this disease. Monday morning I was concerned because I had been so thirsty, had drank so much and had been peeing a lot, so I went to visit my favorite internist and told her I was sure I had diabetes. A quick blood test later confirmed my blood sugar was about 49 (normal), and that instead, what I suffered from was too much heat, too much water, too much tea, and too much hypochondria. The internist told me to exercise and lose weight—and I did lose some weight. I figured that golfing was good enough exercise—alas; as I have grown older, I have discovered that a bit of exercise does actually make me feel better. I wish I had started that program sooner—but that is another story.

High Blood Pressure

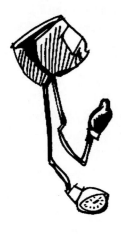

If your little heart has to pump blood to an extra hundred pounds it might need to increase the pressure it uses to pump that blood. Furthermore, the narrower the arteries become because of atherosclerosis (not just those to the heart), the higher your blood pressure must be to deliver the same amount of blood to your body.

Think of it this way: if you have a garden hose delivering water to your plants and you kink the hose, the pressure in the tube goes up and you have to have more pressure to deliver that same water. But, if you deliver water at a higher pressure to that garden, you will disrupt the garden a bit— you have to be gentle with the garden (at least that is why I think Mom didn't want me running through hers).

The same goes for organs like the kidneys, the eyes, or the brain—the higher the blood pressure, the more damage is done. Just like to mom's garden, you need to water it, but you have to water it at a pressure that won't disrupt the plants. High blood pressure delivers blood at a pressure that will cause damage to the organs that receive it, like the heart, kidneys, eyes, or brain. High blood pressure can lead to strokes, blindness, kidney failure, as well as heart attacks and impotence. So, get your blood pressure under control and be gentle when watering the garden. Strokes are one of the leading causes of deaths in the United States, and the elimination of obesity will greatly reduce the risk of strokes.

Cancer

There have been many studies showing that people who are overweight (obese) have a higher incidence of cancer than those who are not. Part of the problem comes from the fat cells themselves; besides storing fat, they are also your body's warehouse for hormones, toxic chemicals, and a few other things. The more storage space you have the more stuff you store that can cause cancer cells to be stimulated. People with cancer who starve themselves tend to live longer than those who eat a lot. The first evidence of this came from victims of concentration camps: some of the individuals who went into concentration camps had been diagnosed with cancer and while in the camps were in remission. Upon being liberated from the camps, when they resumed their normal diet, their cancer recurred. Starvation is not recommended as a treatment of cancer, however. Research about obesity and cancer is in the early stages. Other studies out of Harvard have shown that diets rich in high-glycemic index carbohydrates cause a higher incidence of cancer.

Research has shown that 14 percent of cancer deaths in men and 20 percent of cancer deaths in women may be due to excessive weight. One study speculated that 90,000 cancer deaths could be prevented if America simply slimmed down. Obese males are four times as likely to die from cancer of the liver, and obese women have six times the death risk from cancer of the uterus. Obese people are also at risk for cervical, ovarian, non-Hodgkin's lymphoma, stomach, liver, prostate, multiple myeloma, and several other types of cancer. Almost every type of cancer has been studied and a startling fact emerged. There are more obese patients with cancer than not.

Cirrhosis of the Liver or Fatty Liver

There is a condition called fatty liver, also known as non-alcoholic steatohepatitis (NASH), or its newer name, non-alcoholic fatty liver disease (NAFLD) which is associated with obesity. This occurs when there is a build up of fat in the liver. While fat in the liver is not a problem, it can cause an inflammatory response and ultimately can lead to cirrhosis and even death from liver failure. The build up of fat in the liver of patients with obesity is not related to fat in the diet, but rather to a diet rich in carbohydrates (again, common cause of obesity in the United States). It is also highly associated with Type II Diabetes and patients with elevated blood triglycerides (both related to obesity).

Fatty liver can occur in patients who have had the obesity surgery called the jejuno-ileal bypass. This surgery is no longer performed, partially because there were a number of deaths from liver disease. The modern surgeries, which are performed for weight loss, including Roux-en-Y gastric bypass, duodenal switch, vertical banded gastroplasty, and the lap-band, have not been associated with this complication.

Weight loss surgery can reverse the fatty infiltration of the liver. If fatty liver goes unchecked, it can lead to cirrhosis. As a side note, one reason The American Society of Bariatric Surgery recommends that individuals who have had the jejuno-ileal bypass have it reversed is because of the incidence of fatty-liver.

Just to add to this trauma, if you are morbidly obese, you are not a candidate for a liver transplant or any other transplant.

High Cholesterol and High Lipids

—or, how to keep the blood slick

Just about everyone has his or her cholesterol level and lipid levels checked these days. Elevated levels of blood cholesterols are not a good thing and can lead to heart disease. Elevated levels of triglycerides also can lead to disease of the heart and blood vessels. The elevated levels of the various forms of cholesterol and lipids form a complex group of diseases with a genetic component, and if yours are elevated you should talk with your physician about getting these levels under control. The most often advertised drugs in the United States are medications designed to decrease the blood levels of cholesterol and lipids. Weight loss will also decrease blood levels of cholesterol and lipids and may lower them enough that you no longer need that expensive medication for them. While some diets claim that avoiding fats will lower cholesterol, and other diets say avoiding carbohydrates will lower cholesterol, no one disputes that getting rid of excess body weight will lower your cholesterol and lipid levels. Cholesterol and lipids are the things that cause those nasty plaques on the blood vessels and these lead to heart attacks, strokes, kidney failure, and other diseases.

Sleep Apnea

—snore, stop, snore some more

Sleep apnea is a condition that causes people to stop breathing for periods of time when they are sleeping. Apnea is another fun Greek word, meaning "without breath." Being breathless when your romantic partner sees you is great, but when it comes to sleeping, if you want to wake up rested, it is better to breathe. There are a number of types of sleep apnea, but they are all related to obesity, and sleep apnea can be a source of obesity all by itself! There are three types of sleep apnea: obstructive, central, and mixed. Obstructive is when part of your airway flops down and obstructs your ability to take a breath while sleeping. Sometimes as you take a breath, it comes as a snore. Central apnea is the lack of a signal from the brain to breathe, and "mixed" is a combination of the two. All types may be cured with weight loss. When you stop breathing at night your brain wakes you up a bit so you take a breath. This leads to a long restless sleep.

Sleep apnea causes restless sleep and can lead to high blood pressure, memory loss, narcolepsy, poor attention span, heart problems, impotency, and an overall sense of not being well-rested. It is responsible for automobile accidents, as victims of it may fall asleep at the wheel of the car while driving.

Some people develop sleep apnea when they reach a certain weight. There are treatments for sleep apnea, so if your partner thinks you snore a bit too much you should be tested. A number of patients with sleep apnea syndrome are cured within several months following weight loss surgery. A good night's sleep makes you feel more energetic the following day, and with more energy, you can exercise and lose more weight. Your metabolism will be higher the day after a good night's sleep—again promoting weight loss.

People with a BMI >27

- 56% have high blood pressure
- 47% have elevated blood cholesterol
- 70% have Type II Diabetes

Joints

—they were not designed with this weight in mind

A number of patients come to bariatric surgeons because they need a hip or knee replacement and the orthopedic surgeon refuses to perform it as long the patient is morbidly obese. Even if you don't need a new hip or knee, imagine your entire weight on a joint. Losing weight is a great way to keep your joints healthy as long as you can. Besides, walking feels better if you don't have as much weight on the joint.

Pseudotumor Cerebri

This is a condition where the brain has a bit too much spinal fluid in it, and because of obesity, it cannot release it. This can cause severe loss of function, blindness, headaches, and a number of other problems. Weight loss will cure this in many cases.

Obesity-related problems that don't limit your life, but make it miserable:

- joint problems
- heel spurs
- heartburn
- urinary stress incontinence
- leg swelling
- varicose veins
- tight airline seats
- tight everything seats
- heavy or absent menstrual periods
- poly cystic ovarian disease

Other Fun Things

-not necessarily co-morbid but major pain in the neck

Obesity is associated with a lot of other things that can make your life miserable but that are not considered "co-morbidities." These things cannot kill you, but they can make your life miserable. They are all related to obesity and all improve after weight loss.

(a) Heel spurs – A condition that makes it painful to walk. The heavier you are, the more weight you put into every step. As you lose weight and walk more, these improve. Sometimes heel spurs require surgery, but often your friendly podiatrist can treat them with some inserts for your shoes.

(b) Stress incontinence – Your bladder spills urine when you laugh or sneeze. The more weight you have on your bladder from your belly, the more pressure there is on the bladder. Losing weight not only decreases that pressure, but also reduces your risks should you require surgery for stress incontinence.

(c) Heartburn – Some people notice that they have heartburn when they reach a certain weight. Pregnant women notice that heartburn goes away after delivery of their newborn and returns once the newborn becomes a teenager! The weight in the abdomen puts pressure on the diaphragm and increases heartburn. Some patients will still require medicine for heartburn or acid production, but weight loss decreases this problem for many patients.

(d) Swelling of the legs – Swelling of the legs and ankles has a number of different sources, as do all of these conditions. There is no doubt that decreasing the amount of weight on your legs and ankles diminishes the swelling.

(e) Tight airline seats – Some of my patients can't travel anywhere unless they buy a first-class seat. They are just too uncomfortable in those small airline seats. Losing weight makes it much easier to sit in those airline small seats although the food is still better in the front seats.

(f) Polycystic ovarian syndrome (PCOS) – Patients with this problem have difficulties with their cycles, have multiple ovarian cysts, and some have over production of certain hormones that cause excess facial hair on women.

(g) Infertility – Some women have difficulty becoming pregnant because of obesity. The first line of treatment, your gynecologist will tell you, is to lose weight. As with PCOS, there are a lot of hormonal changes when someone is morbidly obese. Even as patients lose weight, the hormones fluctuate quite a bit. Most bariatric surgeons recommend that patients wait two years after weight loss surgery to become pregnant.

(h) Varicose Veins – Okay, I admit it—I am Norwegian, and my Norwegian medical textbook defines Varicose Veins as veins that are too close together. Varicose veins are caused by a backward flow of blood. As the blood pools in the veins, they slowly enlarge and those nasty spider veins develop. This can be unsightly, but it can also cause you to have tired legs at the end of the day, your feet can swell, and you may feel tenderness over the veins. Excess weight definitely contributes to this problem.

All these conditions are aggravated by obesity. As people lose weight, these conditions are much easier to control and some disappear entirely. Some insurance companies will designate these as "co-morbidities" of obesity, but most will not.

Major Disclaimer Here

Skinny people die young. Skinny people develop diabetes, cirrhosis, sleep apnea, joint problems, heart disease, infertility, heel spurs, and all the rest. We all know skinny people with bad hearts. We all know thin folks who have diabetes. Weight loss will certainly eliminate a source of problems, but it may not eliminate the problem. I have plenty of patients who no longer need medicines for high blood pressure or diabetes—and many patients who need less medicine than before. While I don't think of weight loss as a cure for diabetes as one of my colleagues does (I tell patients they still have that predisposition), but it sure is a lot easier to avoid problems by losing a hundred pounds.

1-23

One of my favorite patients was a very nice young man named Fred. When he came to me, he weighed over 560 pounds and had a problem with congestive heart failure. Fred went home and lost 100 pounds within the first six weeks. Unfortunately, he died of heart failure a bit later. He was happy to be getting around better, and was a wonderful inspiration to a lot of people in my support group. Surgery can help you lose weight, but it cannot cure the damage caused by years of obesity or the underlying diseases.

Who Cannot Have the Surgery?

Weight loss surgery is elective, meaning you can plan the time of the surgery. It is not an emergency like that for a ruptured appendix. Most people who decide this surgery is for them want the surgery today or tomorrow. After an article of mine was published in a local paper, I was called to the hospital to do an emergency consultation for weight loss surgery—kind of funny if you think about it.

Some patients are too ill to have the surgery. It is sad when obesity plays a major role in the heart disease or other problems these patients suffer from, but sometimes these diseases are too far advanced to make surgery a safe option. When I have patients like this I feel sad because, had they been referred for weight loss surgery sooner, they could have avoided the ravages of obesity.

Sometimes patients may need other medical procedures prior to weight loss surgery—for example, if they need their heart stented or bypassed, this is better done before obesity surgery (heart beats guts like rock beats scissors).

Some surgeons refuse to operate on patients who continue to smoke, and some even go so far as to do random testing of blood for nicotine. It may seem a bit odd to some people, I realize, but I am one of those who will not operate on smokers. There are several reasons for this. The main reason is that smokers have a higher incidence of problems following surgery, including pneumonia, leaks from the anastomosis (more about this later), as well as hernias. We even make our patients sign a contract that they will quit smoking and it has been quite successful. It's a great way to change a few bad habits and choose life over obesity and smoking.

Psych Evaluation

Many insurance companies and bariatric surgeons require patients to have a psychological evaluation prior to undergoing weight loss surgery. Some patients simply are unable to comply with the changes they will need to make, are unable to understand, or they have compulsive eating behaviors that need treatment. A number of patients have clinical depression, which is not cured by weight loss surgery, and it may even be exacerbated by the surgery. Patients with depression need to be on medication for a month before undergoing the surgery. A lot of my patients get a bit nervous about seeing a psychiatrist or psychologist before the surgery and ask me what it is all about—I tell them it's just routine, just not to tell about the voices they hear. However, psychological issues are important and I became a firm believer after meeting Larry—unfortunately.

Larry was the nicest fellow you could imagine. He came to my office and consulted with me about weight loss surgery. He was so happy that there was an answer to his obesity. He also had Hepatitis C and had not been treated for it, so we arranged treatment prior to surgery. He was a thoughtful fellow and sent me a card—through e-mail—and thanked me for not judging him for his obesity. Four days later, he committed suicide. Not only was I shocked, so was my staff—because he didn't display any signs of depression. I don't know if I should have felt honored that he thanked me in his suicide note or ashamed that I didn't see his underlying depression and send him off to see the psychiatrist. Depression is very common among patients with obesity, but there is medication to treat it. If you are depressed, please see someone, please!

Age is a factor with obesity also. While there is a chapter about obesity in young folks in this book, older people often ask about weight loss surgery. I worry that obesity might have already done irreparable damage to older people by the time they get to me, but I have to tell you about Dottie. Dottie is about the nicest person you could ever meet. She was 63 years old when I met her and in great health—we even had her undergo some heart tests. She loved the support group and adopted all of my patients as her children. She lives many miles away from Phoenix, she said, because she lives on a fixed income and can't afford to live in a big city. To pay for her trips to the monthly support groups, she makes jewelry and sells it—she is quite talented, I might add. I was hesitant to do her surgery, but she sailed through like a champion, and at her one-year anniversary had lost 135 pounds and felt great. Sometimes age is more than a number. Not only am I so happy that we operated on Dottie, but my support group does a lot better when Dottie is there to give us all hugs.

You really need a support system after you have this surgery. You need to belong to a support group, believe it or not, and there is more about that later in this book. More importantly, you need someone who can be supportive during this process. Some patients don't want friends or family to know about their surgery and that is fine. That is your business, but you do need someone to help you through it.

Everyone worries about their ability to comply with the life changes weight loss surgery requires. They come to us because they have failed countless diets and weight loss programs. They have tried the funny little machines to lose weight, or even have had liposuction before and these have failed. The vast majority of people will be successful with a weight loss surgery program, but some will not. Contrary to a popular, slightly overweight, psychologist, it isn't psychology or willpower that causes obesity, it is biology. In surgery we change your biology and a strange thing happens: patients feel full with less food and that gives them a sense of control over food that they never felt before. Not that there isn't a bit of willpower involved, and not that you won't be on a diet for life, because you will. But guess what—most of my patients lose more weight than the surgery is designed for them to lose. Why is that? Is it because I am a great surgeon, or that I have a 100-watt smile? No (okay, I really want to take credit, but the smile is because of Crest), it is because they have far more willpower than their skinny sister-in-law or the pop-television psychologist ever gave them credit for. All those diets you lost weight on—remember those? Those proved you had willpower. Remember, we change the biology and all of a sudden you can lose weight.

You really need a support system after you have this surgery.

So, worry about it but recognize that once your guts are rearranged, so is your life—forever. That can be a good thing, but it can also be a bad thing, depending on your attitude. You have to know what you are getting into.

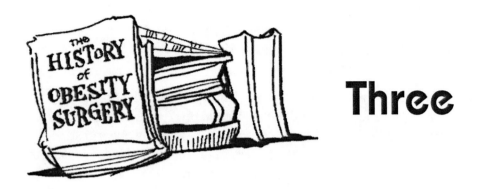

Obesity Surgery History

Obesity: It Is a Disease

We have all seen the Metropolitan Life Insurance Company standards that have the "ideal" body weight. These were initially determined in a height/weight category by simply noting that there was an increased death rate among people who had certain height/weight ratios. But, society, as well as industry and most of the medical profession, did not consider obesity to be a disease. Surgeon, J. Howard Payne first coined the term "morbid obesity" in an attempt to convince insurance companies there was a level at which obesity became a disease, and that there were some surgical treatments for that disease. Those surgical treatments were based upon years of clinical observation and trials.

The field of weight loss surgery is called "bariatric surgery," which always sounds like we are diving—and sometimes we think we are.

History of Weight Loss Surgery

Gee, you don't need this but here it is anyway

Surgeons are keen observers of their patients. We have fat ones, skinny ones, all kinds. But when someone who once was fat becomes skinny, we pay attention to what we did.

So it all started with an observation—that patients who have less small bowel get skinny. The small bowel (made up of three sections: the duodenum, jejunum, and ileum) is the major "absorptive" part of the intestine. Some patients, for a variety of reasons, loose a portion of their small bowel. Okay, they don't lose it; some very nice surgeon has to remove the small bowel. If a lot of small bowel is removed (more than 80 percent) the patients are given the diagnosis of "short bowel syndrome." Patients with short bowel syndrome are a challenge, and before the days when we could give them nutrition through an intravenous line, many of these patients died of malnutrition. The idea then was that if you bypassed a lot of the small bowel on purpose, the patients would lose weight.

The most common and popular weight loss surgery in the 1960's and 1970's was the jejuno- ileal bypass. Essentially, you bypassed all but a foot and a half of the twenty feet of small bowel. Many patients found that they could eat anything they wanted and still lose weight. It was primarily a malabsorptive procedure that led to rapid weight loss, often one hundred pounds in the first couple of months. Over the long term, however, some patients developed severe complications. Because of these complications, any individual who had this surgery is advised to have the surgery reversed or revised into another weight loss surgery. Liver failure, which led to the death in 91 patients, was the most severe problem, and is the main reason this surgery is no longer offered. Other complications attributed to this surgery include kidney stones, arthritis, and osteoporosis from disturbances in calcium metabolism. The

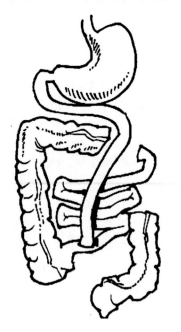

surgery essentially hooked the first part of the small bowel to the colon. This decreased the amount of absorption that patients could have and, in the process, it increased diarrhea and made for some severe disturbances in the electrolytes of these patients.

One famous surgeon spent the first half of his career doing these surgeries and the second half of his career undoing them. Then there was the other problem. After a while, the remaining 18 inches of small bowel accommodated and patients began to regain their weight. This surgery hasn't been done in the United States since the 1980's, although there are still a number of people around who had the surgery. About once a year, most surgeons see a patient who wants a revision to some other form of surgery. So, if you or a friend of yours had the "jejuno-ileal" bypass, we recommend you see your local bariatric surgeon to have that surgery revised.

They noticed that if they removed part of their patient's stomach, the patient could not eat as much and he tended to lose weight.

The next observation came from those surgeons who did a lot of stomach surgery. They noticed that if they removed part of their patient's stomach, the patient could not eat as much and they tended to lose weight. This was a forced "portion control." This began a series of operations whose purpose was to limit how much a person could eat or drink. These are called "restrictive" surgeries. Pure gastric-restrictive surgeries were first started with true "stomach stapling." A staple gun was fired horizontally across the stomach, with a small opening in the middle that allowed a little food to pass through. This operation failed because the upper stomach was able to distend easily. One of my favorite hospitals in Phoenix was a pioneer in this stomach stapling procedure, doing 12,000 of them over time. This surgery was ultimately replaced with the vertical banded gastroplasty (VBG), which is a much better surgery.

These surgeries, and variations of them, are mentioned because both can easily be revised to another type of weight loss surgery. Revision of surgery is offered to patients who have had either of these surgeries.

The Bad Old Days Tainted Weight Loss Surgery

These early surgeries gave bariatric surgery a bad name. Some of the prejudice against weight loss surgery can be traced to these procedures that either failed early on, or had significant morbidity and mortality (our surgical term for complications and death) for their patients. Some insurance companies deny patients payment for either a long-limb Roux-en-Y gastric bypass or the duodenal switch, thinking that the malabsorptive part of the surgery is reminiscent of the jejuno-ileal bypass. There is a great deal of prejudice against weight loss surgery among physicians. Often patients come to my office after begging their primary care physician to refer them for a consultation for weight loss surgery.

Surgical history is filled with stories about unsuccessful, at the least, or deadly early attempts at the first surgery. Cardiac surgery is an example: today coronary artery bypass is almost "routine surgery," but in the early days of cardiac surgery, there were many failures.

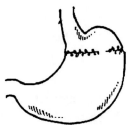

Horizontal Gastroplasty

Stomach surgery is the same. Many of the first stomach operations led to death and all surgeons know the name of the first man who successfully operated on the stomach in 1881 (Bilroth—a Swedish surgeon who worked in Vienna).

The National Institutes of Health and Weight Loss Surgery

Bariatric surgery continues to evolve and many careful and thoughtful surgeons continue to develop surgeries and watch their results. The most famous is Iowa surgeon Dr. Mason, who not only developed and perfected a couple of surgeries, but also followed patients and encouraged other surgeons to follow their patients to see the long-term effect of surgery for weight loss.

But obesity and weight loss surgery, were also watched by a group of scientists and physicians who were brought together by the National Institute of Health to form "consensus" statements. These are "non-advocates," meaning that the members of this panel were not advocating any particular surgery, but merely gathering the research and facts at that time to make a determination bout obesity and surgery. There was a 1978 consensus statement that showed concern for the jejuno-ileal bypass, which was ultimately abandoned.

Major Consensus Statement

The NIH's major consensus statement was released in 1991. Among their findings, the panel recommended the following:

(1) Patients seeking therapy for severe obesity for the first time should be considered for treatment in a non-surgical program with integrated components of a dietary regimen, appropriate exercise, and behavioral modification and support.

(2) Gastric restrictive or bypass procedures could be considered for well-informed and motivated patients with acceptable operative risks.

(3) Patients who are candidates for surgical procedures should be selected carefully after evaluation by a multidisciplinary team with medical, surgical, psychiatric, and nutritional expertise.

(4) The operation be performed by a surgeon substantially experienced with the appropriate procedures and working in a clinical setting with adequate support for all aspects of management and assessment.

(5) Lifelong medical surveillance after surgical therapy is a necessity.

It is also useful to quote them:

Patients whose BMI exceeds 40 are potential candidates for surgery if they strongly desire substantial weight loss, because obesity severely impairs the quality of their lives. They must clearly and realistically understand how their lives may change after operation.

In certain instances less severely obese patients (with BMIs between 35 and 40) also may be considered for surgery. Included in this category are patients with high-risk co-morbid conditions such as life-threatening cardiopulmonary problems (e.g., severe sleep apnea, Pickwickian syndrome, and obesity-related cardiomyopathy) or severe diabetes mellitus. Other possible indications for patients with BMIs between 35 and 40 include obesity-induced physical problems interfering with lifestyle (e.g., joint disease treatable but for the obesity, or body size problems precluding or severely interfering with employment, family function, and ambulation).

Back to surgery

What were they doing?

Soon the jejuno-ileal bypass surgery was gone and various surgeons were working on their own version of weight loss surgery. The majority of those efforts are seen in the drawing.

I will go over the various surgical options available today. Some are simple variations of another and will not have much to say about them. Suffice it to say: Surgery is a well-studied option for obesity. bariatric surgery continues to evolve. Newer surgeries such as the lap-band (introduced to this country in 2001 and to Europe in 1993) and duodenal switch (used since 1988 in this country) are two of the latest versions. The widespread use of laparoscopy to perform weight loss surgery has decreased the hospital stay and improved laparoscopic skills among many of the surgeons in this country. No doubt, in the future, as the biology of obesity is better understood, we will develop other procedures perhaps in conjunction with better medication for weight loss.

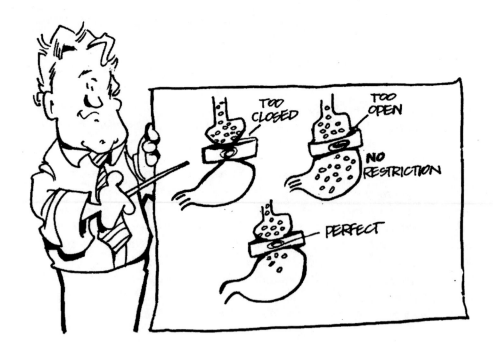

The Future of Weight Loss Surgery

Pacemakers and Balloons

There are two new tools on the horizon for weight loss surgery. One is the Gastric pacemaker where, during surgery, some electrodes are placed on your stomach and a battery is implanted under your skin. This device works, so they say, by decreasing your appetite. It is not yet approved by the FDA and is currently in trial in the United States. The idea is appealing, but the results are not as good as another minimally-invasive surgery—the lap-band. Both require the same sort of surgery, but the pouch for the battery is larger than the pouch for the lap-band port. Electrodes have to be periodically replaced at a far higher rate than the tube for the lap-band. Weight loss for the pacemaker has yet to equal the lap-band, but the results are for early trials.

Remember the balloons placed in the stomachs in the 1980's? They had a few problems, like sometimes they would deflate and cause a bowel obstruction, so they are no longer used. The idea was a good one, however. A balloon in the stomach made you feel full so you ate less. Well, building on that idea, a new device is being developed and a new trial will be underway. The idea behind this balloon-like device is to use it as a temporary measure for people who have a lot of weight to lose, such as those in the super-morbidly obese class. Losing some weight prior to surgery will allow them to have a safer surgery. If we can bring a patient from a BMI of 60 down to one of 45, the risk of surgery decreases substantially. Could this be used for the last 40 pounds or so? Maybe, but that is not the intent.

A variety of adjustable laparoscopic bands are used in Europe and the rest of the world. The only approved band in the United States is the lap-band manufactured by Inamed. These other bands will be arriving once they have undergone FDA trials. For example, Johnson and Johnson anticipates their band will be ready for market in 2007. There is no evidence that any of these bands are better or worse than Inamed's lap-band.

How Dr. Terry Re-arranges the Guts

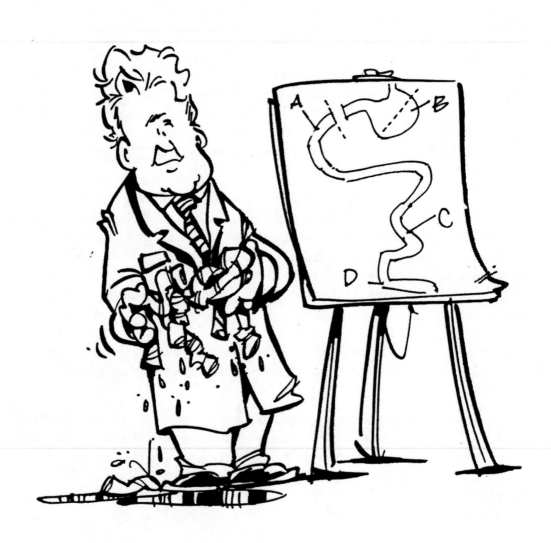

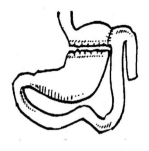 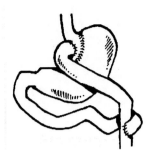 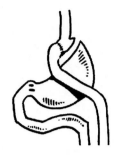

Gastric Bypass with Loop Gastro-Jejunostomy **Gastric Bypass with Lesser Curve Pouch and Roux En-y** **Transected Roux-En-y**

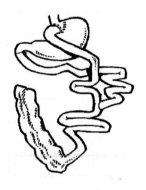 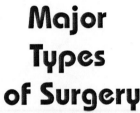 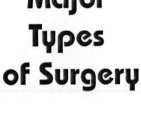 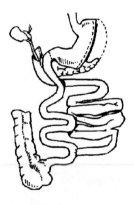

Major Types of Surgery

Long-limb RNY Gastric Bypass

DS Surgery

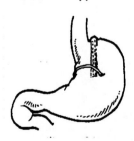 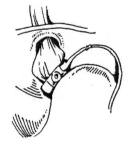 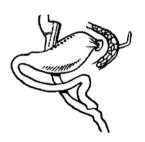

Silicone Ring Vertical Gastroplasty **Adjustable Lap-band** **Fobi Pouch**

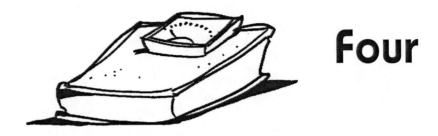

Four

Why People Need WLS

There is nothing complicated about obesity. Fat is nothing more than storage, and some people have abundant storage! To get fat you must eat more calories than you use. Calories come in delicious forms, many of which are highly condensed. In surgery we simply change the way the digestive system works. In all surgeries we limit the amount of food you can take in, and with some surgeries we make the guts a little less efficient at digesting and absorbing calories.

Obesity or Smoking—Which is Worse?

If you are a cannibal, don't eat the smoked ones

With 27 percent of the American population defined as obese (BMI >30) you have to wonder why. There is plenty of blame to go around, and you have no doubt heard it. Of course, the trial lawyers are going to become involved with a class-action lawsuit against fast food places, but they are like vultures, picking off the corpulent carcasses of our citizens.

Smoking is clearly a problem and smoking—ask any addict—is one of the hardest addictions to quit. But America is doing it. The percentage of Americans who smoke has gone down over the years. Once, the majority of Americans smoked. Now the smokers are in the minority. We mobilized Americans against smoking. Why not obesity?

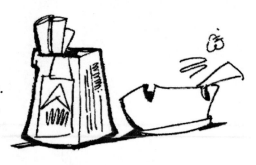

Eating is not an addiction. Eating is necessary for life itself, so reducing the amount of food consumed is possible, but giving up food is not. The latest trend with fast food restaurants is encouraging as they are providing alternative meals that have fewer calories, less fat, and are more nutritious. A few years ago, it was hard to imagine going to *Jack in the Box* for a good salad, but that is what people are now doing.

Super Size It, Please

When I was growing up in Alaska we didn't have a McDonald's but I loved going to Oregon where my grandparents lived because my brothers and I could walk the six blocks to the McDonald's on 82nd Street. I thought hamburgers were better than pot roasts back then. Now I wish that my grandmother were alive to make me a roast.

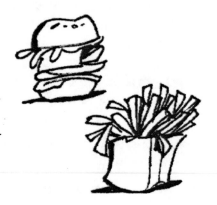

Ten years ago, McDonald's had a sale on their hamburgers. You could buy the 1964 hamburger for the 1964 price of a quarter, so I did—and I couldn't believe how small it was. Then, of course, I ordered a proper quarter-pounder, fries, and a coke (for a few cents extra it was super-sized).

The simple lesson here is this: the portions Americans eat have increased over the years, and as our meals have become larger, so have our belt sizes—after all, we do clean up our plates. The burgers are bigger, the bagels are bigger, the pizza is larger, and there are more fries in a serving. And have you seen the size of the soda containers? I had goldfish bowls smaller than those!

The secret is in the packaging. It isn't too expensive to throw in a few more fries or add some extra soda and people don't mind spending a few more dimes for the larger size. Apparently, the founder of McDonald's thought that if people wanted more French fries they would simply buy more—but they didn't. People hardly ever go back for seconds. One of his employees, who had been in the movie theater business, suggested the super-size concept, and it worked. It costs just a few cents to put a few more fries in, and customers think they are getting a bargain. This concept has caught on and all of the fast food places are doing it.

"Restrictive" surgeries combat overeating—super-sized meals will no longer fit in your stomach. All weight loss surgeries have a restrictive component.

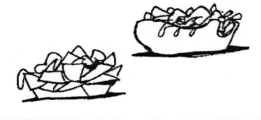

As the standard of living in other countries increases, so does their tendency toward obesity. You can find super-sized portions all over the world. The concept has gone beyond fast food places to local restaurants. Even in the Middle East I was told I could have a few more slices of swarma for some extra Euros. Most of us have been taught to clean our plates; it is almost un-American, or un-world, if we don't.

Part I – The Stomach Side of WLS

The way Mother Nature put our guts together makes a lot of sense. The way we surgeons re-arrange guts also makes sense. There are two broad categories of weight loss surgery: "restrictive" (or "portion control") and "malabsorptive" (or "bypassed").

All weight loss surgeries have some restrictive components to them. The purely restrictive surgeries are the adjustable laparoscopic band and the vertical banded gastroplasty. All surgeries allow you to feel full, or "satiated" with smaller quantities of food.

VBG	Lap-band	RNY	Duodenal Switch	BPD
Restrictive only	Restrictive only	Restrictive and malabsorptive	Restrictive and malabsorptive	Restrictive and malabsorptive

There is no pure "malabsorptive" surgery. The last one was the jejuno-ileal bypass, and that did not work well. Surgeries with a malabsorptive component include the Roux-en-Y bypass, the duodenal switch, and the biliopancreatic diversion. These surgeries do not actually cause "malabsorption." Instead, some of the small bowel is bypassed so that it becomes less efficient at absorbing food. The increased success of these surgeries is directly related to the malabsorptive component. In fact, the higher the BMI of the patient, the better they do with a longer bypassed limb.

How We Restrict the Super Sizes

The stomach regulates a lot of what we do in bariatric surgery. Surgeons make the stomach smaller so that it cannot hold as much food. Every operation does this differently. The most radical operations are the "micro-pouches," which are a version of the Roux-en-Y gastric bypass that reduce the capacity of the upper pouch to about one-half an ounce. The larger pouches are found with the biliopancreatic diversion, which hold 8 to 9 ounces. The BPD is rarely done in the United States, as most surgeons prefer the duodenal switch, which is the "upgraded" model.

Pouch size for various weight loss surgeries

VBG	Lap-band	RNY	Duodenal Switch	BPD
1 ounce	1 ounce	1/2 to 1 ounce	4-8 ounces	8-9 ounces

The job of the stomach is to reduce the size of food particles so they can be expelled into the small bowel and be more easily digested. The stomach does this by producing acid, which helps break things down, and an enzyme called pepsin. Once the food particles are 1-2 millimeters in size, they are expelled into the duodenum through the pylorus. If they cannot be broken down, they may remain in the stomach for a long time and form bezoars or be vomited. Bezoars are formed from material that is too large to be expelled and cannot be broken down into smaller pieces.

When the stomach is distended, a signal is sent to your brain that you are full, and that the stomach needs to empty. This signal is a complex mechanism involving several hormones. Ghrelin is a hormone that is manufactured by cells in the stomach, and it is released when the stomach is empty. When Ghrelin levels are high, you feel hungry. After a meal, the levels become quite low. Obese patients have low levels of Ghrelin that are attributed to chronic eating. In patients who have undergone gastric bypass surgery, Ghrelin levels are also low—which means these patients feel satisfied and full.

The simple goal of surgery on the stomach is to make you feel satisfied with less. The longer food is kept in the stomach, the longer you are satisfied. Certain foods do not remain in the stomach for a long period of time, such as liquids, high-carbohydrate breads and potatoes, and other soft mushy foods. Foods that remain in the stomach longer and produce a feeling of "satiety" (or not needing more food) include proteins, such as meat, fish, and poultry, as well as low-glycemic carbohydrates, such as lentils, beans, most vegetables (except potatoes) and fats. The more fiber there is in a carbohydrate, the longer it appears to keep you satisfied (of course there are always exceptions).

How We Keep Food in the Smaller Stomach

VBG	Lap-band	RNY	Duodenal Switch	BPD
Small stoma, reinforced so it cannot be enlarged	Small stoma, adjustable	Small stoma, constriucted to be about 1/2 inch	The pylorus, the normal mechanism	Small stoma, constructed to be about 1/2 inch
Silicone Ring Vertical Gastroplasty		Stoma-		

The operations help to keep food in the stomach as long as possible. Normally this job is done by the pylorus, which regulates when food or liquid may leave the stomach. The duodenal switch operation is the only operation that allows this normal mechanism to remain in place. This is one of the advantages cited for those who perform this surgery. As with most of surgery, the more you can maintain a normal anatomy, the better—hence, the duodenal switch allows for a more normal food intake, a more normal mechanism for satiety, and allows patients to have fibrous foods, all of which cannot be said for the other weight loss surgeries.

For the RNY and BPD the anastomosis, or opening between the stomach and small bowel is made small during surgery. The inner diameter of this opening (or stoma) is about 1/2 inch. If it becomes larger than this, then food passively leaves the stomach into the small bowel and no feeling of satiety is generated.

The analogy is an hourglass. If you make the opening between the top of the hourglass and bottom of the hourglass larger, then the hourglass empties quicker. The same thing happens with the stomach—the larger the opening, the faster the food empties, and the quicker you feel hungry again.

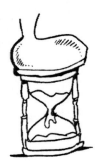

The advantage of the lap-band is that the surgeon can adjust the size of the stoma, allowing for maximum feeling of satiety. In people who need more nutrition, like women who become pregnant, we can open the stoma to allow in more nutrition.

For all weight loss surgeries, the types of food that can overcome the sensation of fullness are the same: mushy foods, milkshakes, potatoes, breads, and pastas. Essentially, no operation will overcome high-glycemic index carbohydrates. The mantra of *"protein first"* is essential in all surgeries in order to maintain a sense of fullness.

"It's the Carbs, Barb"

–said a ten-year post op patient

Barbara Metcalf, RN, has been working with obese patients for many years. One patient had a duodenal switch ten years ago, lost over 120 pounds, and maintained a weight between 160 and 170 pounds. The only time she regained weight was when she was laid up after a leg fracture, but she lost that forty pounds quickly. She finds that she can maintain her desired weight easily, as long as she monitors her carbohydrate intake. Even for duodenal switch surgery, which maintains the most normal of the stomach digestive process, carbohydrates can cause weight gain, and limiting them promotes weight loss.

The success of weight loss surgeries depends upon ensuring that you feel full for a long period of time. Surgeons help ensure that success by constructing the pouch to be small and by making the opening into the digestive system small. The patient is responsible for the rest of the success by eating a diet that will remain in the stomach, or pouch, for a long period of time (these include proteins and low-glycemic index carbohydrates).

Normal Digestion

Digestion takes place when bile and pancreatic juice (coming from A and B) mix with food in the duodenum after leaving the stomach through the pylorus (C).

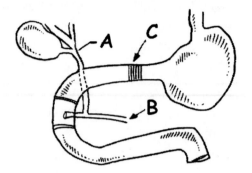

The food in the stomach is expelled into the duodenum through the pylorus (also known as "the holy pylorus"). The stomach's job is to mix things, allow the acid to break them down, and begin the process of digestion. Once the material has a certain consistency it is allowed to make the journey through the pylorus. The pylorus, labeled "C", is a sphincter that allows liquids and small particles of food though, but not large particles and not dense solutions (they have to be diluted a bit).

Leaving the pylorus, the food enters the duodenum, one of my favorite places in the body. Into the duodenum comes bile, which is made by the liver. Bile assists in the breakdown of fat. Bile empties into the duodenum (the bile duct is labeled A) two to three inches from the sphincter (labeled C). The gallbladder is simply a storage unit for bile, if you don't have the gallbladder your liver simply makes more bile—people live quite well without the gallbladder.

The pancreas also empties juices into the duodenum (the pancreatic duct is labeled B). The pancreas makes a lot of fluid that helps to neutralize the acid of the stomach. If the acid of the stomach isn't neutralized, an ulcer might result. The most common place for an ulcer is in the area just after the pylorus, above the pancreatic duct—which makes sense. The acid first hits here and the pancreatic juice to neutralize it comes in a couple of inches later. The pancreas also secretes powerful enzymes to help break down protein. So when the contents of the stomach mix with the contents of the duodenum, there is more digestion of food. These digestive juices work all through the bowel to breakdown food into smaller and smaller particles that can be absorbed in the small bowel.

All bypass operations separate the stomach contents from the bile and pancreatic juice. Again, the VBG and lap-band do not fall into this category; their sole mechanism is to restrict food intake—or portion control. The point where the stomach contents rejoin the duodenal juices is called the common channel. The longer the common channel, the more digestion occurs.

Part II – the "Bypass" Part

Limiting absorption by limiting the common channel

The distance between the stomach contents and the contents of the duodenum (which contain the digestive juices of the bile and pancreas) determines whether we call the procedure a distal bypass or a proximal bypass. In the original, factory-installed digestive system (normal anatomy), the entire small bowel sees both the food and the bile and pancreatic juices. This would equate (in our medical terminology) to a "common channel" of about six yards. That makes for very efficient digestion.

The Details

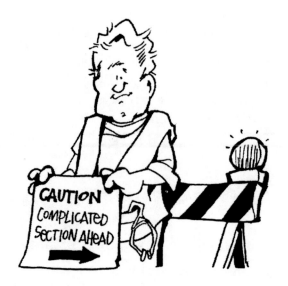

This chapter contains technical details about how the guts are rearranged to make various distal bypass procedures–the Distal RNY, the Duodenal Switch, and the BPD.

The plot is quite simple—they all start as distal procedures and we rearrange the small bowel the same way for all of them. It is what we do to the stomach during the operation that makes the difference. If you want to see how we do this, read on and follow the gut diagrams. If not, take my word for it and skip to the Q and A section at the end of this chapter.

Distal Versus Proximal Bypass

The length of the bypassed segment determines whether it is called a distal bypass or a proximal bypass. If we bypass 10-15 percent of bowel it is a proximal bypass. If we bypass more than 50 percent, then it is a distal bypass.

The difference between a proximal bypass and a distal bypass depends on where we cut the small bowel. As you can see from figure A, if we cut it at point A it is a distal bypass, and if we cut it at point B it is a proximal bypass.

The first step in any distal bypass procedure is the same. All distal bypass procedures follow the steps described below.

Figure A

First the small bowel cut 200 centimeters from the colon (or about 40
percent of the length of the small
bowel) cut at point A.

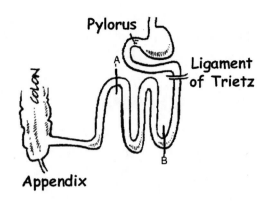

Figure B

This leaves two limbs of the
Roux-en-Y (RNY). The one limb will
be attached to this small bowel where
the "attach here" arrow is pointing.

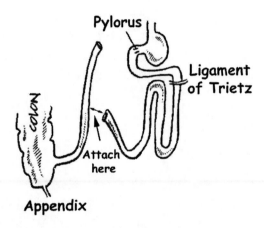

Figure C

Here the limb is reattached—form-
ing a "T", although we like to say it
is a "Y", where that Y is is called the
common channel. In this example the
common channel is made about 100
cm long.

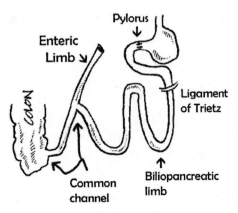

Figures A, B, and C represent the steps for the duodenal switch, the BPD, and the distal RNY gastric bypass. Technically, all of these operations are a long limb RNY bypass. The difference between them is what we do to the stomach.

Duodenal Switch

The most common distal procedure is the duodenal switch. To do the DS we need to do everything in Figures A, B and C.

The first step in the duodenal switch is to make the long limb Roux-en-Y bypass (figures A, B, and C). The difference with the DS is what we do to the stomach.

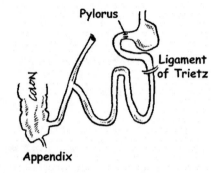

In the DS we cut a portion of the stomach and send that to pathology. We also make a cut an inch from the pylorus.

The old stomach is sent away. The long-limb of the Roux-en-Y is attached to the first part of the duodenum. The other side of the duodenum is sewn closed.

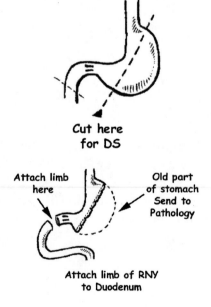

Now we attach everything and this is the final product.

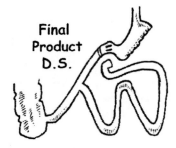

So, as you can see, the duodenal switch is merely a Roux-en-Y bypass below the first portion of the duodenum.

Biliopancreatic Diversion

The biliopancreatic diversion has been largely replaced by the duodenal switch. There are still places that do this operation, so we put it here for completeness.

Again the first step to making the BPD is to make the long-limb RNY bypass (Figures A, B, and C). The difference is that with a BPD, we make the common channel shorter (50 cm instead of 100 cm). The other difference is what we do to the stomach (see below).

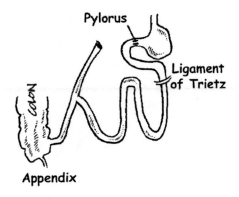

We cut the stomach in two places. The upper stomach is about 250 cc or 8 to 9 ounces.

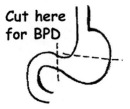

The lower stomach is completely removed and the duodenal stump is sewn
over. The RNY will be attached to the
large pouch.

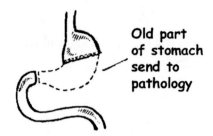

Old part
of stomach
send to
pathology

Unlike the DS, the common channel
for the BPD is 50 cm, or 20 inches.
Again, the BPD has largely been
replaced by its "upgraded" model,
the duodenal switch, which allows
a more normal digestion with the
pylorus in place, doing its job.

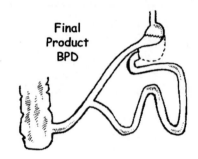

Final
Product
BPD

The BPD and the standard Roux-en-Y gastric bypass do appear similar,
however the differences are worth noting. The BPD has a 9-ounce pouch and the
lower stomach is completely removed. With the standard gastric bypass there is
a one-half to one-ounce pouch and no stomach is removed.

Distal Roux-en-Y Gastric Bypass

To make a distal RNY gastric bypass, we
divide the stomach into a one-ounce upper
pouch.

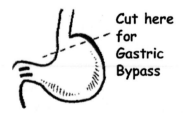

Cut here
for
Gastric
Bypass

With the two parts of the stomach we will attach the limb of the RNY to the upper pouch.

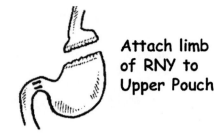

Attach limb of RNY to Upper Pouch

This final product is a distal RNY. Again, the common channel is 100 cm. In this configuration, the duodenal contents and also some of the stomach juices go through the duodenum, but not food.

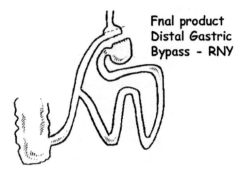

Fnal product Distal Gastric Bypass - RNY

The typical "proximal" gastric bypass has a Roux-en-Y limb of 50 to 60 centimeters, and it is reconnected about 15 centimeters from the ligament of Treitz (with an average of 75 cm of bowel not seeing either food or duodenal juices). This means that the common channel, where duodenal contents and stomach contents meet, is about 525 cm. In terms of "malabsorption," this is essentially none. If we lengthen the bypass from 75 cm to 150 cm (thus shortening the common channel to 450 cm), there is a noticeable difference in patient outcomes.

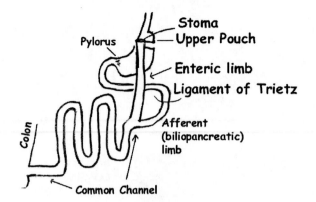

This is a proximal bypass, where the afferent or bioliopancreatic limb is 15 cm and the enteric limb is 60 cm, for a total bypass of 75 cm. The common channel is 525 cm long.

Longer limb bypasses tend to have more weight loss. We call these procedures "malabsorptive." The distal surgeries used today (DS, distal RNY) produce only "moderate malabsorption." Why is it that patients with higher BMIs (>55) tend to lose more weight with distal procedures? The answer is simply by limiting calories. By creating a shorter common channel, we limit the amount of calories absorbed. Primarily, we are limiting the absorption of fat.

This does not mean that only higher BMI patients should have distal bypass procedures. The primary mode of weight loss for all surgeries is restricting the amount of food you can eat. The small bowel becomes more efficient at digestion as time goes on so, no matter how short your common channel is, over the course of years it will absorb more fat and calories.

Frequently Asked Questions

Should only patients with a BMI >50 have distal bypass procedures?

No, all obese patients can benefit from distal bypass procedures. It is an individual choice between you and your surgeon. While restricting intake is successful for weight loss, a longer bypass can lead to better, more sustained weight loss.

Can there be too much bypassed, or too short a common channel?

Yes. Most surgeons limit the common channel to no shorter than 100 cm (40 inches). If you have a shorter channel you can develop protein-calorie malnutrition. Some patients benefit do from shorter channels, but the concern is always that they may not absorb enough protein. Again, this is the choice of the surgeon.

Can there be too much malabsorption?

Yes, which is why the common channel size is important. With a 100 cm common channel it is very rare to have a patient become malnourished.

Can the common channel lengthen with time?

Often it does. The body does a great job of "accommodating" for shorter lengths of bowel. When re-operating on patients, surgeons often note that the common channel has lengthened.

If the common channel gets longer, can that contribute to regaining weight?

Yes. But typically the common channel should become better at absorbing things as time goes on. Most people regain weight not from the common channel getting longer, but from the stomach (or pouch) increasing in size and patients eating more carbohydrates.

With a distal procedure, I heard I can eat whatever I want and not gain weight. Is this true?

There are always patients who claim they can eat whatever they want and still maintain a normal weight. This is a misperception on their part. There is no surgery that will allow that. You must always have protein first when you have distal bypass procedures and if you do not, you will become ill.

Why can't I have a purely malabsorptive procedure?

The jejuno-ileal bypass was just that. There was no limitation with the stomach. Many patients thought this was ideal, as they could lose weight and eat what they wanted—or so they thought. Over time, however, these patients regained weight. Restricting intake is an essential part of weight loss surgeries, and one of the most important building blocks of all bariatric surgeries.

What is the main cause of weight regain after weight loss surgeries?

The main cause is eating too many high-glycemic index carbohydrates. The most common finding of patients who have regained their weight is that the stomach size has increased (or pouch size).

How does the stomach (or pouch) get larger?

Typically this is done by constantly challenging it with increasing quantities of food. This is why we stress measuring your food before eating it. The stomach does not become larger by overeating at one single meal. Measuring twice and eating once is better than chronically overeating.

What are the advantages of the VBG and Lap-Band over the bypass surgeries?

The purely restrictive operations require fewer supplements than do the bypass operations. All patients who have undergone weight loss surgery should be taking vitamins (in fact the National Academy of Science recommends that all adults take a daily vitamin). With the VBG or lap-band you probably will not need supplemental iron, vitamins A, D, E, K, or Vitamin B12 supplements. The purely restrictive surgeries tend to cause constipation, whereas the long-limb bypass operations tend to cause loose stools.

Can a proximal bypass be converted to a distal bypass and visa versa?

Yes, this can be done. More often the proximal bypass is converted to a distal by pass when the patients are not losing enough weight. But the common channel can be lengthened if patients aer having severe malabsorption or problems with diarrhea.

How do I choose the right operation for me?

There is no magic formula. Choose the operation that your surgeon does as a matter of routine. Some insurance companies will only cover certain surgeons or certain operations. They all work for weight loss. Learn all you can about the operation you choose, learn how to live with that operation and how to make your new anatomy work for you. If you are lucky enough to have a choice of surgeons and operations, then choose the operation that appears to work best with your lifestyle. No matter which operation you have, you will eat differently after surgery than you do now.

Can the common channel be too short?

Yes. Not everyone is the same and a 100 cm common channel may not allow enough absorption of bile, protein, or foods, leading to protein malnutrition or severe diarrhea. Some patients may need to have their common channels lengthened.

Couldn't I just have a restrictive surgery and not have a malabsorptive component?

Yes. The major source of weight loss for all surgeries is the restrictive component. The restrictive surgeries are the safest, do not require supplemental minerals, and they allow the entire GI system to be examined with an endoscope.

What will prevent me from shrinking to nothing?

The stomach, or the pouch, does enlarge with time and you will be able to take in more calories. We expect this and want it to happen. Early on you will not be able to eat much, but as time goes on you will be able to eat more. Use this "golden time" to make good food choices.

Major types of surgery for weight loss	VBG	Lap-Band or other adjustable types of bands	RNY Including Fobi Pouch	RNY-distal	DS/BPD BPD without DS is rarely done in the United States
Percent of weight lost at five years	40-60%	50-75%	50-75%	60-75%	>75%
Ranking for weight loss	4th	? (1 or 2)	3rd	2nd	1st
Vitamins needed	Yes	Recommended	Yes	Yes	Yes
B12 needed	No	No	Often	Often	Occasionally
Calcium needed	Rare	Rare	Recommended	Yes	Yes
Iron needed	Sometimes	Rare	Often	Often	Often
Foodrestrictions	Chew well	Minimal	Fiber may cause bezoars. Dumping may occur with high carbohydrates	Low fiber, High protein	No restrictions. No dumping
Downside of this operation	High compliance needed for success	Requires adjustments	Dumping, ulcer formation, strictures	See RNY. 3-4 stools per day. Increased vitamin ADEK deficiency. Foul smelling flatus	3-4 stools per day. Vitamin ADEK deficiency. Foul smelling flatus (gas)
Upside to this operation	Minimal long-term nutritional problems.	Safest of all surgeries	Best studied of all operations, most commonly performed	Good combination for patients with BMI over 50	No abnormal food restrictions.

Following Surgery

No matter which surgery you have, here are a few simple things you will observe afterwards.

1. It won't take much to make you feel full, and that is just fine.

2. Don't let a friend or family member tell you to eat more. Let that be between you and your bariatric surgeon. If you should eat more, your bariatric surgeon will tell you.

3. You will find that kid-sized meals are more than you need.

4. Appetizers are great sources of protein and are the right portion size for you.

5. Use a smaller plate and smaller utensils (forks, spoons) so you mentally redefine a portion size.

6. Meals can be planned much better than snacks. Eat three meals a day so you do not feel the need to have a snack. Snacks tend to be high-calorie items, in contrast to meals that can be nutritious.

7. If it takes you longer than 45 minutes to eat, you might be grazing, and grazing is one sure way to defeat any weight loss operation.

8. You can eat more if you drink and eat at the same time (with the RNY)—so don't. Learn to chew well.

9. Hey, spending 19 cents on a burger is better than two bucks, and you will have plenty to eat.

10. There are few bad foods, but there are bad quantities of foods.

Those ten points are just a preview of what is coming up for you.

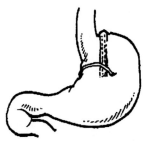

Silicone Ring
Vertical Gastroplasty

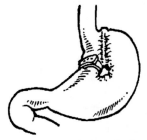

Vertical Banded
Gastroplasty

Five

The VßG Surgery

The Vertical Banded Gastroplasty (VBG) is a pure restrictive operation that simply works by restricting the intake of solid food. VBG comes in two forms, the Vertical Banded Gastroplasty and the Vertical Silastic Ring Gastroplasty. These operations are functionally the same but have one minor difference; the material used to reinforce the stoma.

Like Sands Through the Hourglass

–so are the calories of our life...

The stomach is surgically altered to act as an hourglass, where the upper stomach holds about one ounce and the food drips into the lower stomach at a rate dependent upon the size of the stoma (or opening between them) and the thickness of the food. Solid food takes longer than puree or mushy types of foods. This stoma is reinforced with a band of material made of either

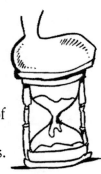

Marlex mesh (VBG) or a silastic ring (VSRG). The band material (either Marlex or silastic) is the only difference between these operations. The band does not stretch, meaning the stoma cannot be enlarged by constantly challenging it with either more food or larger food particles.

Once food is eaten, it slowly drips into the lower pouch through its stoma (or the opening between the upper and lower pouch). When this small amount of food is in the upper pouch, a feeling of fullness (satiety) is present, creating an enforced "portion control."

As with most weight loss surgeries, the feeling of fullness (satiety) is one reason for the success of this operation. Patients develop a sense of control over food, often for the first time in years. A change within the brain occurs, and I would only be speculating if I told you it was in the thalamus or the cortex, or any other brain parts—suffice it to say that there is more to appetite control than satiety.

It Isn't Fun to Vomit

Overfilling the pouch leads to vomiting, as does putting something into the pouch that cannot go through the stoma (a large piece of meat, some vegetables, some fruits—bananas are a common offender). This reinforces control over the amount of food eaten. However, some discover that some foods go down easily, especially those dense in calories such as milkshakes, mashed potatoes, donuts, potato chips, and other high-calorie snacks. This can reinforce negative eating habits, lead to eating foods that "go down" easily, and override the procedure.

Some people are more likely to have trouble with the VBG than others. You may have trouble if you:

- have dental problems leading to an inability to chew food thoroughly
- consume a large concentration of calories coming from a liquid source
- eat lots of sweets
- have a history of bulimia (induced vomiting for weight loss)
- demonstrate an unwillingness to change habits
- need to take a lot of pills

A diet history is important in determining if the VBG or lap-band would be an appropriate surgery. If you cannot keep away from "soft," high-carbohydrate foods, then this procedure is not likely to benefit you.

Requirements following VBG:
- fully chew food before swallowing
- not drink liquids while eating
- have the ability to stop eating when full
- avoid high calorie liquid items
- take a multivitamin daily

Highly suggested changes to maximize VBG benefits:
- exercise at least 45 minutes four times per week
- take nutritional classes to maximize meal planning
- avoid snacks
- avoid "soft foods"

Advantages of the VBG:
- no blind segments of the digestive tract
- no dumping
- no calcium deficiency
- no protein malnutrition
- minimal monitoring of vitamin and minerals
- allows endoscopic and radiologic evaluation of the GI tract

Disadvantages of the VBG
- less effective than the RNY for sustained weight loss
- less effective as a weight loss procedure for control of diabetes
- requires implantation of a foreign body (marlex or silastic)
- behavior changes important for long term success

Note: Patients who are in the "super" morbid obese category benefit less from this procedure.

While this is a relatively simple operation, it still has all the risks of any bariatric procedure. However, newer stapling instruments have improved some outcomes and decreased the incidence of breakdown of the staple line. This procedure is well suited to a laparoscopic approach. At one time, this was the most popular bariatric procedure, but it has recently decreased in popularity—perhaps because of studies showing better results with the RNY gastric bypass.

An entire industry was built around the VBG surgery, with a hospital group that put together the Life Lite program. This program brought patients from

The VBG is a fundamentally sound procedure and has been performed extensively in the bariatric community.

around the country to a few major centers where the silastic ring VBG variant was performed. This program was later dismantled, although it had developed its own stapling device and training program for its surgeons. Surgeons now run their own bariatric programs in individual hospitals. Recently the pendulum has returned to where surgeons are joining a larger association of physicians or hospitals, ostensibly for marketing purposes.

The adjustable laparoscopic band (ALB), such as the lap-band, is replacing the VBG in some areas. Recently, some newer laparoscopic techniques for the VBG have led some prominent surgeons to prefer the VBG over the ALB. What they lose in doing this, however, is the ability to adjust the band over time.

The main disadvantage of both the lap-band and VBG is the behavior modification requirements for success. This bariatric surgery, more than the others, requires patient compliance. Unfortunately, there is no test (psychological or otherwise) to help determine which patients would benefit from this procedure over other procedures. Experienced surgeons have a difficult time determining which patients would benefit from this procedure. Patients who follow-up with support groups and aftercare clearly do better than those patients who do not.

This procedure can later be revised to another procedure if necessary, a distinct advantage. Some believe that VBG can be revised to a RNY much easier than a lap-band to the RNY. However, this may simply be their lack of experience with the lap-band. Most surgeons note that the lap-band is not that difficult to remove.

The VBG is a fundamentally sound procedure and has been performed extensively in the bariatric community. When the jejuno-ileal bypass was abandoned as a weight loss procedure, most patients were converted the VBG. It was determined to be a safe, reliable procedure with minimal long-term complications, and became the staple of bariatric surgeons for a number of years. It continues to evolve in terms of laparoscopic techniques and some believe that the adjustable laparoscopic band may have evolved from it.

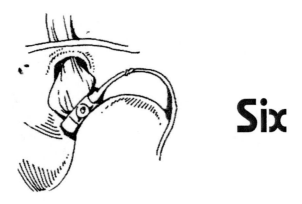

Six

Adjustable Lap-band Surgery

The adjustable laparoscopic band is the latest and the safest surgery for weight loss. Currently, only the lap-band (manufactured by Inamed) is approved in the United States. During the operation the surgeon places an adjustable band around the stomach, creating a small upper pouch. This pouch initially holds about one ounce or less, so it doesn't take much food to fill up a patient. The early feeling of fullness leads to portion control, and the decreased caloric intake leads to weight loss. As time goes on, adjustments can be made to the stoma to facilitate weight loss, or it can be opened to allow more nutrition. Surgeons noted years ago that when they removed the distal portion of the stomach, patients lost weight. Using the band to divide the stomach into these two sections decreases the amount of food the distal stomach "sees" and weight loss occurs.

The lap-band is widely used in Europe and was approved for use in the United States in June 2001. Over 14,000 have been placed in the United States in the first two years after approval. Ozzy Osbourne's wife had this type surgery, and she is a clear example of how successful this surgery can be. If your spouse is considering having this done, we highly recommend a recording contract.

The surgery takes an hour or so and is done through a laparoscope. The band is placed around the upper part of the stomach, and the inside of the band is a balloon. A small bit of tubing connects the port (reservoir) buried in the chest wall with the balloon on the band. A surgeon can place saline (saltwater) in the port, which inflates the balloon. By filling the balloon, the band tightens and the opening between the upper and lower stomach (known as a stoma) narrows. The surgeon can add saline, or remove saline, from the band to adjust the opening size quickly and easily right in his office.

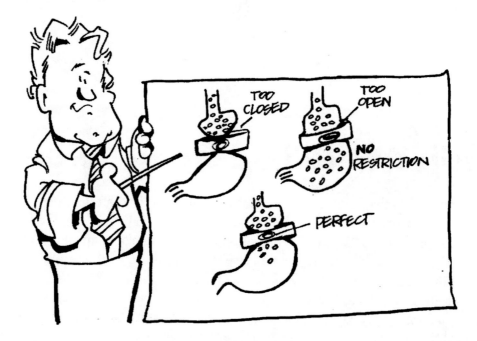

Typically, when the band is initially placed in the patient, it is not filled at all. It is usually placed loosely and is allowed to scar in place for several weeks. Once the band is secure, the surgeon then does a "fill," or inflates the balloon to narrow the stoma and provide restriction. Patients typically go home the day after surgery, and even though the band is loosely placed, most patients notice that they feel full with a lot less food right away. Four to six weeks after the band is placed, the surgeon does the first "fill." With this fill, the patient feels restricted and begins to lose weight. As they lose weight, they also lose some of the fat around the stomach so further fills are needed to maintain a restriction.

Weight loss occurs because a patient feels full with a small amount of food, which stays in this upper pouch. The stomach becomes like an hourglass, similar to the VBG, and the food drips into the lower stomach at a rate dependent upon the size of the stoma and the consistency of the food. Liquids drip out of the pouch quickly, whereas solid foods take a bit of time to drip into the lower pouch.

There are several other advantages of the ALB. It is the least invasive surgical option, there is no intestinal re-routing of the guts, the operative time is an hour or less, and there is less patient pain, hospital stay, and recovery period. Proponents of the ALB also cite fewer peri-operative and post-operative complications. In North America, during tests, one of the largest series had no deaths associated with the lap-band.

Some doctors consider this a good solution for obese teenagers since there is no malabsorption of nutrients.

Some doctors consider this a good solution for obese teenagers since there is no malabsorption of nutrients. It is also recommended for patients who are at very high risk for surgery. Because patients can easily absorb medications after this type surgery, these surgeries are preferred for transplant patients who are very dependent on absorption of their medicine. There is no dumping syndrome nor its related dietary intake restrictions. The bowel is not entered into or cut with the lap-band, so intestinal leaks are less of a problem than with the VBG.

If a woman becomes pregnant, the surgeon can remove the saline from the port, deflating the balloon and opening the stoma. This allows the increased nutritional needs of the fetus to be met. Maria became pregnant two years after her band was placed. The stoma was opened and she had a very healthy boy. Shortly after delivery, the band was re-inflated so she could lose the 90 pounds she gained during pregnancy. All weight loss surgeries are safe for pregnant women with close monitoring by the peri-natologist (fancy OB doctor who watches high-risk pregnancy). As with all weight loss surgeries, we recommend that women wait to become pregnant for at least two years after surgery.

> **The following patients might benefit more than others from the Adjustable Laparoscopic Band:**
>
> - patients whose serious attempts to lose weight have resulted in only short-term success
> - patients who do not have any other disease that may have caused them to be overweight
> - patients who are prepared to make major changes in their eating habits and lifestyle
> - patients who are willing to continue working with the specialist who is treating them
> - patients who do not drink alcohol in excess

The bad wrap the lap-band has received is due to its high revision rate. Revision means that the patient has to go back to surgery to change the position of the band in cases where it slips or needs some adjustment. In some centers, this rate of return to the operating room was reported as high as 17 percent. Now the company has drastically changed training requirements for surgeons in the lap-band system. For example, surgeons who wish to be trained with the lap-band must show that they are skilled with advanced laparoscopy. The surgeons are also "proctored" by an experienced surgeon. While this may seem excessive, since it is a fairly simple procedure, sometimes a few tips from an experienced surgeon will save revisions later. Even experienced surgeons will sometimes have to revise a band.

The early published results of the lap-band in the United States were not similar to the results in Europe. However, that has changed. The lap-band now has weight loss results that are similar to other surgical procedures. Some centers have better results than others. Excess weight loss of 61 percent at two years is the average.

Other companies are submitting their adjustable laparoscopic band for FDA approval. Companies such as Johnson and Johnson's Ethicon division will no doubt recruit surgeons who have appropriate surgical-laparoscopic abilities to beta-test it, and require a commitment to follow-up with the patients. There is no reason to believe that one system is better than another is, although it is a possibility. Over 100,000 lap-bands have been placed worldwide, with results published in more than 500 publications. Many surgeons use this as their only weight-loss method. Lap-band surgeons point to the advantage that this surgery is "reversible." While this is the most reversible of all weight loss surgeries, this surgery should be chosen on its merit, not reversibility.

The lap-band can be overcome by eating "mushy" foods, such as mashed potatoes, milkshakes, breads, and the like. These high-carbohydrate foods are easy travel quickly out of the upper pouch, not producing a prolonged sense of "satiety" and contribute to weight gain. These same high-carbohydrate foods will cause failure in all weight loss operations. However, if the patient follows the pre-scribed diet (like the one found later in this book), this surgery is very successful at keeping off excess weight. Eating high protein foods, or low glycemic index carbohydrates leads to more weight loss, as they produce a prolonged feeling of satiety.

Some surgeons leave the lap-band in place and divert the first portion of the duo-denum (a hybrid DS type of operation). There are no long-term studies of this operation. If a lap-band procedure fails, then the cause of that failure must be examined before modify-ing it to another operation. If the cause of the failure is technical and the band needs to be revised, then revising to another procedure or simply replacing the band is appropriate.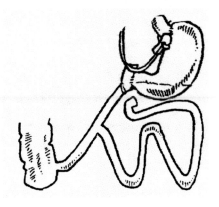

If the failure is secondary to non-compliance, such as a patient consuming too many carbohydrates, then the patient's ability to comply with the required diet needs to be evaluated before a surgeon converts a patient to another proce-dure. No surgery can solve the behavior problems of grazing, consuming high-carbohydrate foods, or drinking milkshakes.

Some feel that the lap-band is the ideal bariatric surgery. The surgery is fast, often taking less than an hour. Recovery from the surgery is fast, with most patients going home the following day and returning to work within a week. There is no intestinal re-routing, and therefore no malabsorption, and minimal requirements for vitamins. The adjustable lap-band is the most common weight loss surgery in Europe and Australia and may become the major weight loss surgery in the United States.

Insurance companies seem to have difficulty with this procedure—some call it "experimental" or "investigational." It is neither. The FDA approved this procedure in June of 2001, and it has met the test of safety and efficacy in the United States. Furthermore, it also meets the criteria of the 1991 National Institute of Health Consensus statement:

Among their findings, the panel recommended that (1) patients seeking therapy for severe obesity for the first time should be considered for treatment in a non-surgical program with integrated components of a dietary regimen, appropriate exercise, and behavioral modification and support, (2) gastric restrictive or bypass procedures could be considered for well-informed and motivated patients with acceptable operative risks, (3) patients who are candidates for surgical procedures should be selected carefully after evaluation by a multidisciplinary team with medical, surgical, psychiatric, and nutritional expertise, (4) the operation be performed by a surgeon substantially experienced with the appropriate procedures and working in a clinical setting with adequate support for all aspects of management and assessment, and (5) lifelong medical surveillance after surgical therapy is a necessity.

Gastrointestinal Surgery for Severe Obesity. Proceedings of a National Institute of Health Consensus Development Conference. *March 25-27, 1991. Bethesda, MD. Am. J Clin Nutr. 1992 55 (2 Suppl): p. 487S-619.*

As you can see from point number 2, the adjustable laparoscopic band clearly fits the definition of the NIH consensus statement.

Going Out of the Country for Your Surgery

While this procedure is slowly gaining approval from insurance companies, many patients may need to pay cash for this procedure and it may be less expensive to have it done outside of the United States. The band itself is expensive (currently selling for over $2995). In addition, with hospital fees, the surgeon fees, anesthesiologist fees, the total cost of this band placement can be $15,000 in the United States. It still costs less than most new automobiles and, unlike a car, you will carry your body with you everywhere you go for the rest of your life.

The high cost of medicine in the United States has forced some people to go to foreign countries where health care costs less. This can be a problem, because the key to this procedure is the follow-up and the "fills" that need to be done by an experienced surgeon. Before going out of the United States to have a band placed, make certain you have a surgeon who is willing to do "fills" for you in the United States. If you don't, you should plan on returning for fills outside the U.S. where you had the band placed.

If you have a band placed, you should ask for the patient booklet that comes with the band and the sticker that identifies which band you will receive. The day after your surgery, you will have an upper GI test—ask for a copy of that x-ray and bring it with you to the surgeon who will be following you in the United States.

Some feel that the lap-band is the ideal bariatric surgery. The surgery is fast, often taking less than an hour.

Some adjustable laparoscopic bands have not been approved in the United States. It would be difficult, if not impossible, to find a surgeon in the United States who will agree to adjust those bands.

If you need an adjustment in the United States, often the first fill will be done in x-ray with a radiologist and the surgeon. This may cost a bit more, but this way they can see where it was placed and make certain the band is in the right position. Subsequent adjustments may take place in the surgeon's office.

If you have your lap-band placed outside the United States, you should do the following:

- Find a surgeon who has an associate in the United States willing to adjust the band for you

- Only have lap-bands placed that are approved for use in the United States

- Ask if your surgeon will travel to Mexico to place your band. This allows a good follow-up .

- Take the patient information book and the "sticker" which has the band information with it (lot number, size of band) with you. You might also ask for a copy of the operative report.

- Take a copy of the post-op barium swallow with you

- Expect that your first fill will be done in x-ray, which may cost more than your follow-up fills done in the office.

Some hospitals outside of the United States are every bit as outstanding as those in the states. In fact, some of the surgeons in Mexico and Australia have far more experience than many in the United States.

Band Fills

The band is filled with saline (saltwater) either in the doctor's office or in x-ray. The surgeon's fee for a band fill ranges from $150 to $300. If radiology is used, that may cost an additional $300 or more. The advantage of having the band filled in the radiology suite is that you have rapid restriction of the band instead of having a gradual filling of the band in the doctor's office. Every surgeon has a different protocol for band fills, different time schedules and use different procedures. There is no one right way. After the band is filled, you are placed on liquids for the next three days and then you will go to solids—this gives the stomach a chance to get used to its new anatomy. Eating right solid food too soon after a fill may cause severe discomfort.

Things That Can Go Wrong

Band Slips

The band is loosely placed around the upper part of the stomach, and then a few sutures are used to secure the band in place. If some of the stomach slips underneath the band, then you will need to go back to the operating room for an adjustment. As experience with this product continues, slips are becoming less common. However, violent vomiting can cause the band to slip, which is why many surgeons have you on a liquid diet for two weeks following implantation.

Band Erosions

Sometimes the band will erode into the stomach although erosions have happened less often as the suturing techniques have improved. Even if everything is done perfectly, erosion of the band into the stomach can still occur. When this happens, the band must be removed. One doctor with lots of experience in the band, Dr. O'Brien in Australia, advocates removing the band, sewing up the erosion, and replacing the band immediately. While that flies in the face of what some surgeons would do in the United States, he has had good results. Your surgeon will want to remove your band if it has eroded and allow the stomach to heal before replacing the band.

Port Problems

The port where saline is injected is left underneath the skin of the chest wall. If this port migrates out of the skin or develops an ulcer—call your surgeon. Sometimes this means a band has eroded into the stomach and sometimes it is simply an infection. It is easier to take care of these problems earlier rather than later.

Who Is Not a Candidate?

You may not be a candidate for the adjustable laparoscopic band if:

- you have an esophageal motility disorder.
- you have another disease that makes you a poor candidate for surgery.
- your esophagus, stomach, or intestine is not normal (congenital or acquired).
- you are pregnant. (If you become pregnant after the bioenterics® lap-band® system has been placed, the band may need to be deflated. The same is true if you need more nutrition for any other reason, such as becoming seriously ill. In rare cases, removal may be needed.)
- you are addicted to alcohol or drugs.
- you have an infection anywhere in your body.
- you cannot or do not want to follow the dietary rules for this procedure.
- you are allergic to materials in the device.
- you cannot tolerate pain from an implanted device.

In addition, some surgeons disqualify patients who have a "sweet tooth."

These are relative contraindications, meaning there are always exceptions to these rules. Check with your surgeon first.

A Tool for Weight Loss

The adjustable laparoscopic band is one of the newer weight loss systems available. Like all other surgeries, it represents a tool for weight loss, not a total solution. Advocates of the adjustable laparoscopic band have one argument that is difficult to refute—it is easily reversed. Someday obesity will be treated as a chronic disease like diabetes and when it is, we may have drugs that can treat the disease, rendering surgery unnecessary. In that world, it will be nice to have had a surgery that can be easily reversed.

Lies, Damn Lies, and Statistics

Often patients go to a surgeon who advertises that he does the lap-band but whose first choice for a weight loss tool is *not* the lap-band. Some surgeons use a "bait and switch" approach, advertising the lap-band but talking patients into a Roux-en-Y gastric bypass instead.

The statistics used to convince patients to switch are the weight loss figures at the end of a year—and here is where statistics can fool you. A patient said he wanted a duodenal switch, but was also very interested in the lap-band. We went through the pros and cons of both procedures and the patient decided on the duodenal switch because of the statistics. Those statistics are quite true, I told him. Our patients average 82 percent loss of excess body weight in their first year with DS and 61 percent with the lap-band. But, you can lose all your excess body weight with either surgery. After a duodenal switch, there is rapid weight loss because you have had major abdominal surgery and your body needs a lot of calories to heal itself. After lap-band, you have an easier time from the surgery and use fewer calories.

Most patients who have the lap-band begin weight loss after they have their first "fill," six weeks after the band is placed. The duodenal switch has a head start—but this is not a race. The profound weight loss after major surgery comes with a price. It takes at least 12 weeks after RNY, DS, VBG, or BPD before you feel "normal." Which reminds me, does it ever occur to you that psychiatrists are the ones who define normal? I mean, I remember all my medical school classmates who went into psychiatry and it sort of scares me to think that they are now defining "normal."

The bottom line is this: statistics in weight loss apply to a broad population of patients but they may not apply to you. You can lose weight with any weight loss surgery tool. Pick the tool and the surgeon that make sense to you.

Final Thought

A weight loss surgeon had the lap-band placed in Mexico a year ago. Over the course of the year he lost about 120 pounds. Then he did something remarkable: he removed all the saline from the balloon of his lap-band. He used the lap-band as a temporary measure and is now keeping his weight off on his own. If he gains weight he can get it filled again. He not only learned to eat better but learned to know when he is full. If he gains too much weight, guess what? He refills the band. Now that is a successful surgery!

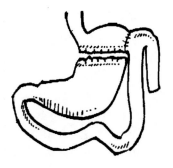

Seven

Mini Gastric Bypass Surgery

The minigastric bypass, first used in the late 1960's and abandoned in the 1970's, was recently brought back because this operation can be done through a laparoscope.

The mini-gastric bypass is very similar to the Roux-en-Y gastric bypass. It functions by dividing the stomach into a small, one-ounce or less, upper pouch from the remainder of the stomach. The upper pouch empties directly into the small bowel.

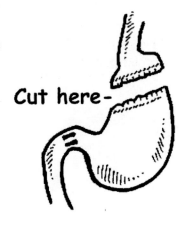

Cut here—

Dr. Simpson's Home Surgery Program

How to Make a Mini Gastric Bypass

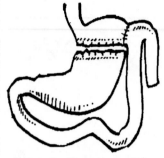

**Gastric Bypass with
Loop Gastojejunostomy**

We bring a loop of small bowel up to the stomach, creating a connection between them in order for food to move out of the upper stomach and into the bowel. This opening between the stomach and the small bowel is called an "anastomosis." That is it—you have now done surgery! Experienced surgeons can do this surgery in about twenty minutes. The short surgery time is one of the advantages touted for this surgery.

How to Make a Roux-en-Y

Now compare the mini gastric bypass surgery to the more popular Roux-en-Y gastric bypass. See the difference? No? There is an extra connection in the RNY that prevents the lower stomach content from moving into (refuxing) the upper pouch.

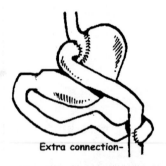

Extra connection-

**Gastric Bypass with
lesser curve pouch
and Roux-en-y**

Why that extra anastomosis? In normal anatomy (anatomy that God gave you, before some surgeon decided to mix it up) the end of the stomach is marked by the pylorus, a one-way valve that helps keep digestive juices out of the stomach.

Food moves from the stomach pouch into the small bowel, (A) also known as the enteric limb. The digestive juices are carried by the small bowel (B) known as the biliopancreatic limb. They join together at C, called the "common channel." The R.N.Y. gastric bypass separates these components of digestion. The RNY gastric bypass diverts digestive juices away from the stomach pouch, avoiding irritation of the stomach by these juices.

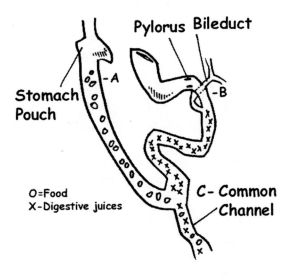

However, as you see in the mini-gastric bypass, those digestive juices, the bile, the enzymes, all flow back into the upper pouch. Normally these juices aren't there and critics of the mini-gastric bypass state that those juices can cause some erosion of the stomach (bile gastritis) and the esophagus.

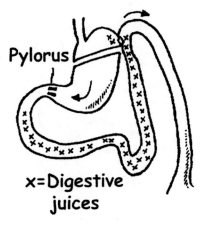

The question remains—is the mini-gastric bypass that bad? It is not supported by The American Society for Bariatric Surgery, nor by a number of insurance companies, but it is fast and it does have the basic components of the Roux-en-Y. The extra connection in the Roux-en-Y serves as protection to the stomach, keeping the bile and enzymes away from it. That extra connection takes some extra time to create and is one extra connection that can leak—although it is rare. The most common connections that leak are the ones between the stomach and the small bowel.

In summary, the mini-gastric bypass was the first gastric bypass done. It was largely abandoned because sometimes the bile and pancreatic juices caused damage to the lining of the stomach and esophagus. When bile refluxes back into the stomach it can cause damage, pain, and ulcers. The mini-gastric bypass does work as a weight loss surgery. The question is whether this is a better procedure than the RNY. The answer is that it is not better. The RNY takes a bit longer to do, but not that much longer. Sometimes it is worth spending an hour or so more in the operating room in order to avoid future problems. Proponents of the mini-gastric bypass surgery say that this surgery works as well as the RNY, and that these concerns are minimal.

So now let us talk about the Roux-en-Y. (Nice segue)

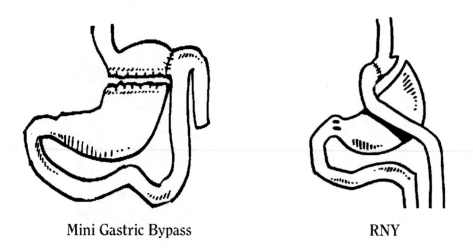

Mini Gastric Bypass   RNY

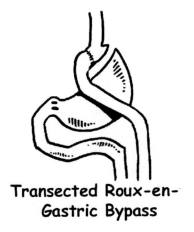

Transected Roux-en-
Gastric Bypass

Eight

Roux-en-Y Gastric Bypass

Roux-en-Y Gastric Bypass (RNY) is the most common obesity surgery done in the United States today. The common names for this obesity surgery are "gastric bypass" or "RNY." Of the 100,000 operations done in 2003 for obesity, 61,000 of them were the RNY type. The other types are lap-band, Vertical banded Gastroplasty (VBG), and the Duodenal Switch.

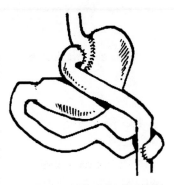

Gastric Bypass with lesser curve pouch and Roux-en-y

Roux, my French friends tell me, means road but this surgery was not named after French roads. Dr. Roux was the name of the surgeon who developed this operation for gastric surgery in 1893.

In RNY surgery, the stomach is completely divided into two compartments—an upper part, or pouch, and the lower portion of the stomach.

Where to cut —

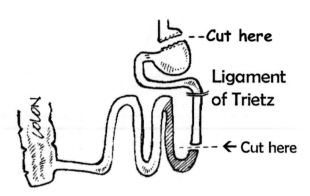

--Cut here

Ligament of Trietz

← Cut here

The upper pouch is smaller, and is made to hold one ounce (about the size of an egg) or less. The small bowel is divided and brought up to the upper stomach where an anastomosis is made between the pouch and the small bowel. An anastomosis is the term surgeons use for the connection formed when they sew or staple together two pieces of bowel, making an opening—or stoma—between them.

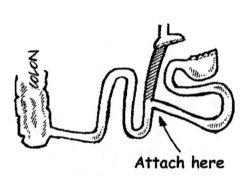

Attach here

Where to connect

The stoma size keeps food in the pouch, allowing the patient to feel full for several hours on a small amount of food.

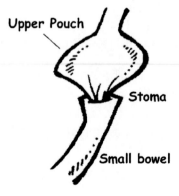

Upper Pouch

Stoma

Small bowel

The anastomosis between the pouch and the intestines is made small so that food will leave the pouch slowly, giving a feeling of fullness. If the stoma is too large, food goes through too quickly and patients don't feel full. If the stoma is too small, then nausea and vomiting may result.

Rules of the stoma – the opening between the stomach and the small bowel:

- If the stoma is too large, you won't feel full
- If the stoma is too small, you will have heartburn, nausea or vomiting
- A meal should stay in the pouch for several hours
- Sip, do not gulp liquids. Gulping can force food into the intestine and you will feel hungry sooner.
- For the first 12 weeks, do not eat and drink at the same time

Since the upper pouch only holds an ounce of food, the patient feels full after eating just a few bites. It is an enforced "portion control" diet. Eating more than the pouch holds can cause nausea, severe discomfort (like you ate all of the Thanksgiving Day turkey) and might lead to vomiting. Learning portion control of food is a difficult task for anyone, but it becomes a way of life after this surgery.

Dumping

Some gastric bypass patients, about sixty percent, develop a syndrome called "dumping" if they eat foods too high in sugar or carbohydrates. Dumping can cause severe diarrhea, cramping, nausea, flatulence, cold sweats, rapid pulse, or a sensation of feeling shaky or faint. This unpleasant sensation can serve as negative feedback and keep patients from resorting to higher-carbohydrate foods. Dumping is not fun—and patients who have this are not happy.

I had one wonderful patient who came to me weighing over 400 pounds. After I did the RNY surgery, he did great, followed his diet, and then, over time, stopped following up with me—as many patients do. He went about enjoying his newer, healthier 155-pound life. Two years later he returned and requested that I do a colostomy (a bag). He said he had such severe diarrhea sometimes that he would wake up at night and be unable to get to the bathroom in time. He had been examined by a gastroenterologist who did a colonoscopy on him and found everything normal. The doctor couldn't understand why this guy had this severe, uncontrolled diarrhea. The mystery was finally solved. He had a lemon tree on his property, and his wife made the best lemonade with sugar. Once his wife started making the lemonade with Splenda®, his diarrhea stopped and she was able to sleep with him again. Splenda is a sugar substitute that does not cause dumping.

Dumping, or the threat of dumping, is one reason some feel that RNY has a better success rate than either the lap-band or Vertical banded Gastroplasty (VBG). Dumping does not happen with lap-band or VBG surgery. Thus, patients who have the VBG or lap-band can drink a lot of high-calorie liquids without dumping. Dumping has no relation to weight loss. You can dump and still absorb sugars and carbohydrates. Dumping can be quite serious, causing blackouts and other severe reactions.

Dumping has no relation to weight loss. All patients experience dumping differently; in the most severe form, some patients find they can never again eat even small amounts of simple carbohydrates like bread, sugar, candy or potatoes.

We have no way of knowing which patients will dump and which will not. So before you choose this operation, know that your days of eating sweets may be over completely. For some this is a desired goal, for others, having an occasional sweet for birthdays or special occasions is a nice reward for weight loss.

Now, if you prefer to have the dumping syndrome because you think it will provide a form of behavior modification, you may be one of the forty percent of patients who will not develop it. Jill was a nice lady with five children who decided to have weight loss surgery because her neighbor had the surgery and it was very successful. She underwent a successful RNY but called me late one night, upset that she was able to eat cookies without triggering dumping. I explained that she was probably one of the 40 percent who wouldn't develop "dumping." She unfortunately continued to feast on cookies and clean her kids' plates. She didn't lose as much weight as her neighbor.

Variations of the RNY

—or, how low do you go

Proximal versus Distal RNY

	Proximal	Distal
Amount bypassed	10-20 percent	Greater than 50 %
Inches bypassed	18-40 inches	More than 120 inches

Normally the small bowel contains a mixture of food and digestive juices. When we bypass a portion of it, some of the small bowel will see food, and some will see the digestive juices, but the only portion that sees both is the common channel. For insurance purposes, a proximal bypass must bypass less than 100 cm (that is, 100 cm of small bowel will not see food). No small bowel is removed.

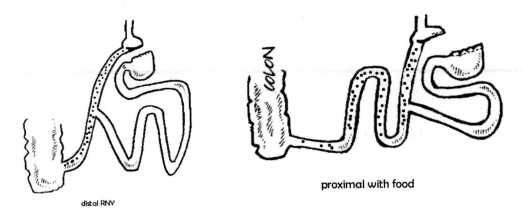

distal RNY

proximal with food

If more intestine is bypassed, another mechanism of weight loss is created called malabsorption. This means, in addition to portion control, there is less intestine to absorb food. Some surgeons reserve the distal bypass for patients who have a BMI above 50, also known as the "super-morbidly obese" patients. Other surgeons use a distal bypass when patients have, through a food history, revealed that many of their calories come from fat.

After distal bypass surgery, patients do not absorb fat as well but they still absorb simple carbohydrates. How much small bowel is bypassed will determine how much fat and complex carbohydrates will be absorbed. Most studies show that a distal bypass can only absorb thirty percent of the fat the patient consumes early on. The reason patients reach their goal weight is not the malabsorption from the small bowel bypass, but from the restriction, or portion control. Over time, the common channel will become more efficient and be able to absorb more fat, protein, and carbohydrates.

There are middle grounds where a shorter amount of the small bowel is bypassed. In these cases less than sixty percent but more than twenty percent is bypassed. There are no rules here for who gets what. Some patients believe that if they have more intestines bypassed they will lose weight faster. But the vast majority of individuals who have gotten to their weight loss goal did it with a proximal RNY bypass. Some insurance companies will deny patients requests to have a "malabsorptive" procedure, calling this "investigational." In 2003 the American Society for Bariatric Surgery, the world experts in weight loss surgery, stated that distal procedures, including the duodenal switch, are acceptable and are not considered experimental or investigational.

As a rule, distal bypass patients have more loose stools, and proximal bypass patients more constipation. But these rules, unlike constipation, are not hard. Each patient reacts differently.

Stomal Stenosis

—or, learning to swallow a big scope

The stoma between the pouch and the intestine is made in a very specific way. Some surgeons use a stapler to make the diameter of the stoma a little less than half an inch in diameter. Other surgeons sew the bowel and stomach together (or make an anastomosis) over a guide so that the size of the stoma will be precise. But as the anastomosis heals, scaring may occur that causes the stoma to decrease in size (a stenosis). When this happens, smaller and smaller amounts of regular food can pass through the stoma and patients develop more vomiting. Your friendly gastroenterologist, or GI doctor, has the cure for this. The GI doctor places a scope down your throat and when it reaches the stoma, he passes a special balloon through it. He inflates the balloon that stretches the scar tissue, and this allows the stoma to open up. Often this needs to be repeated a few times. This is an outpatient procedure, so it may be a bit inconvenient.

Sometimes an ulcer develops at the stoma, resulting in scarring and stenosis (or scarring down in size). Patients with an ulcer need to be on some acid blocking therapy such as Pepcid™ or Prevacid™, and they will also need to have their stoma opened by the balloon dilation. If the stoma becomes too damaged from the scar tissue for the ulcer to be taken care of by a scope, it will need to be revised through an operation. This will require surgical revision, and this means major surgery and hospitalization for a minimum of several days.

How to Defeat the Surgery

The three most common ways to regain your weight...

There are three common ways patients who have the Roux-en-Y gastric bypass defeat the surgery. Defeating the surgery means the patients either don't lose very much weight, or they lose some weight but regain it. The most common mistake is falling back into old eating habits, the habits that caused them to be overweight in the first place. The three most common habits are skipping meals, snacking (or grazing), and eating foods that are high in carbohydrates.

In my seminars, I always ask people to raise their hands if they skip meals—most do. Skipping meals only makes you hungry later and when you become hungry, you will grab the first snack available. These snacks are rarely nutritious and are commonly filled with lots of calories. No weight loss surgery has been invented that is a match for grazing on junk food. Eating a little bit here and there, (grazing) is a great way to get in a lot of calories without feeling full. Alcohol is another source of calories that is often overlooked.

The second most common way to defeat the surgery is to stretch the pouch. We expect the pouch to stretch over time. It will probably stretch to eight or ten ounces after a couple of years, and that is fine. The pouch works by making you feel full with less food. If the pouch stretches and becomes too large, you will eat the same amount of food that you did prior to surgery. That is why it is important to learn what "full" feels like, and why we emphasize measuring your food early in the post-operative process. Many people don't really know what "full" feels like. The feeling of being full (or satiety) often comes thirty minutes after eating (it is kind of a slow reflex). Remember how, after a large Thanksgiving meal, you notice the discomfort 20-30 minutes after eating?

By measuring your food, eating it slowly, and noticing when you are full, you can avoid both pouch-stretch and vomiting. Training your body to notice when you are full, and refraining from eating more food after you feel full, is a goal in the early post-operative period. The pouch doesn't typically stretch after one large meal, but does so from chronically over filling it. The only way reduce the size of the pouch is with surgery, so learn to measure your food early on. The first few weeks after surgery, until they get good at "eyeballing" it, I ask patients to measure everything they eat or drink with a shot glass.

The final way to defeat the surgery is by enlarging the stoma—or opening—between the upper pouch and the intestine. You can cause this by not chewing food well and by forcing large bits of food through the stoma with liquids. Many patients who are at goal weight sip some water with their meal, but they do not gulp liquids. If the stoma enlarges, then food does not remain in the pouch for long and you become hungry.

The only way reduce the size of the pouch is with surgery

Making the stoma smaller often requires an operation. It is a lot easier to learn new habits, like only putting pieces of food in your mouth that are smaller than a pencil eraser and chewing them well.

Don't forget—certain foods stay in the pouch longer than others. These include poultry, meats, and some vegetables. Liquids, soups, yogurt, ice cream, and other soft foods go through the pouch quickly and don't keep you full for long. In fact, most liquids stay in the pouch only a few seconds, moving quickly through the stoma and into the intestine. Some days you can only eat a forkful or two, and other days you can eat more. That is also normal. Just remember— eat slowly, cut your food into small pieces, chew your food well, and enjoy it.

Carbonated Drinks

A real problem or a solution?

Many surgeons do not allow their patients to drink carbonated beverages. There is a little bit of fact here, and a lot of fiction. The facts are fairly simple: most carbonated beverages are very high in sugar or in carbohydrates. Many patients find it hard to give them up, however. I had one lovely lady who underwent the RNY and quickly lost weight, but then she stopped losing for a while. She came back to see me, after having stretched her pouch to over 20 ounces, and wanted a revision. She admitted to drinking about 40 ounces of Coke® a day. I told her once she stopped drinking the cola we would reverse the surgery for her. She never returned.

When you drink carbonated beverages, the concern is that the gas from the carbonation will stretch out your pouch. However, the pouch is NOT an isolated closed bit of stomach. It has two openings, and if you have some gas it will pass one way or the other. Nevertheless, for safety sake—if your surgeon says no carbonation—then do not drink carbonated beverages.

No matter what, **DO NOT DRINK CARBONATED BEVERAGES** for six weeks or longer after your surgery unless instructed by your physician.

Bezoars

Your cat isn't the only one with a hair ball

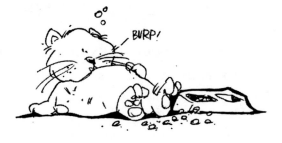

Bezoars are the human equivalent of a hair ball. After gastric bypass surgery some indigestible items can accumulate in the stomach and form a small ball of material which can cause vomiting, a feeling of satiety, weight loss, nausea, and can lead to ulcers or an obstruction.

Bezoars can grow and grow and grow and cause further problems. Small bezoars can pass spontaneously, or with the help of some medications, but most of the time a gastroenterologist will need to either put a scope down and pull them out or fracture them into smaller pieces. Sometimes they are refractory to this therapy and need to be removed surgically. If you develop a bezoar then you have a high likelihood of developing further bezoars.

The four types of common bezoars are: phytobezoars, which are composed of vegetable material; trichobezoars which are composed of hair; pharmacobezoars, which are composed of medications; and lactobezoars, which are composed of baby formula or whey products. For gastric bypass patients, phytobezoars are the most common, followed by pharmacobezoars. Occasionally a bypass patient will develop a lactobezoars, and these are usually patients who are taking whey protein supplements in very concentrated quantities.

Undigested vegetable matter is the most common culprit, which is why a number of surgeons ask their RNY patients not to eat celery, prunes, raisins, beets, persimmons, pumpkins, and grape skins (I like grape skins in the form of wine—they make a zinfandel a nice red color—unless you are like my dad, who prefers white zinfandel, which is made by leaving the grape skins out of the vat). There are a few things that are very hard to digest early on: bananas, oranges, pineapples, and other pulp-laden fruit.

A number of agents cause pharmacobezoars. The most common culprits are antacids, some fiber laxatives, Cholestyramine®, and Sucralfate®, but there are a host of others. Again—just because one pill is good for you doesn't mean the whole bottle is better.

What Happens to the Lower Stomach?

Why your surgeon doesn't want you to take Motrin
The lower stomach is still an active organ. It continues to make gastric hormones, acid, enzymes, and mucous. It does not shrink up or go away. It can also develop ulcers.

The effect of aspirin, Motrin®, or a host of other drugs called non-steroidal anti-inflammatories (NSAID), is to break the protective mucous barrier in the stomach. This does not bother some people too much, but a fair number of individuals end up with some ulcers. While having a pill sit on or in the stomach is irritating, the effect of the NSAID is not dependent on direct contact. This is why a number of surgeons do not like their patients taking these pills (like aspirin, ibuprofen, Naprosyn®, Indomethacin®, and other drugs of this class). If you develop an ulcer in the lower stomach, there is no easy way to have it treated or even diagnosed.

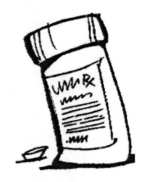

That lower stomach is physically separate from the upper pouch. Normally if a patient develops ulcer symptoms, a gastroenterologist can look into the stomach with an endoscope and make the diagnosis of an ulcer. If that ulcer is bleeding, the gastroenterologist can also treat the ulcer to stop it from bleeding by injecting a drug into it or putting some electric current on the ulcer to coagulate it. These options are taken away once you have a RNY bypass. There is no physical way to get to that ulcer. If these medications are important to your health you might wish to consider some other operation instead of the RNY bypass.

Transection Versus Stapling

How do we separate the stomach?

One other debate among RNY surgeons is whether it is better to physically separate the upper pouch from the lower stomach, or if it is better to staple the stomach sections off from one another but leave them attached. Those who favor stapling without transection note that five percent of patients will break through the staple line, and it is a lot easier to have a patient who leaks into the lower stomach than a patient who leaks into the abdomen, which will make them very sick. Those who transect the stomach into two separate parts state that there is no chance of this leak between upper and lower pouch and that the transected stomach has a lower incidence of leaking than a stapled stomach.

If your surgery is done through a laparoscope, your stomach will be transected. If your surgery is done open it might be done through either one of these approaches.

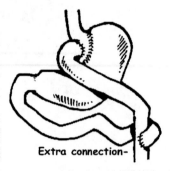

Gastric Bypass with
lesser curve pouch
and Roux-en-y

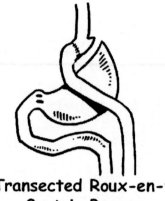

Transected Roux-en-y
Gastric Bypass

Vitamin Supplements for the RNY Patient

Appendix Two contains more details about vitamins and the tests your doctor should order. I want to mention here, however, that patients who have the RNY are subject to iron, vitamin B_{12}, and folate deficiencies. For patients with a long-limb RNY bypass, vitamins A, D, E, and K might need to be added (often drug stores have a pill with those four vitamins in them).

	Multivitamin	Calcium	Iron
Recommended	Daily multivitamin Examples include: Flintstones Centrum Silver Vista	Calcium Daily Tums Citracal	For menstruating women 350 mg a day of iron in either Ferrous Gluconate Ferrous Sulfate Chromagen Forte

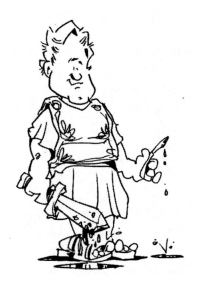

Nine

Duodenal Switch and BPD

An Italian Invention

The duodenal switch operation is derived from the biliopancreatic diversion operation. This surgery was invented by an Italian Surgeon named Nicola Scopinaro. Now I love Italians and all things from Italy. In fact, I've been to Italy twice and I often wonder why anyone would leave such a beautiful place to come to chilly North America—but I digress.

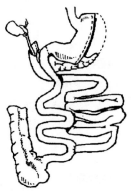

BPD surgery is, for all intents and purposes, a long-limb Roux-en-Y bypass operation. Dr. Scopinaro combined a 65-percent gastrectomy with a long-limb Roux-en-Y. This surgery worked fairly well and was considered to be the most drastic of all weight loss surgeries.

Let us name the limbs of the Roux-en-Y bypass:

- The limb of the Roux-en-Y bypass that has food in it is called the "enteric" limb.
- The limb of the Roux-en-Y bypass that contains the digestive juices (bile and pancreatic juice) is called the biliopancreatic limb.
- Where both limbs of the Roux meet—thus combining the digestive juices with the food—is called the "common" channel.

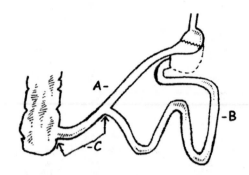

A=Enteric limb (efferent) C=Common channel
B=Biliopancreatic limb (afferent limb)

Okay—now that you have learned some medical lingo, let me give you a couple of other commonly used names. In the Roux-en-Y bypass, the enteric limb is also known as the "efferent" limb (think of enteric and efferent—two e's, or you can think of food exiting—another e, (or you can think of the popular cable channel, but then you would be thinking like the author and would need to have papers to prove sanity). The limb of the Roux-en-Y with the digestive juices is known as the "afferent" limb. You might come across these names somewhere, so I threw them in (just another joy of having bought this book).

If you consider that the common channel in the Scopinaro's operation was reduced to 50 to 100 cm, you can see that this was a drastic step compared with most common channels. In the proximal Roux-en-Y limb, the common channel is 500 cm. The difference accounts for why Scopinaro's BPD operation was successful with weight loss.

All surgeries balance how weight loss is maintained. One component of "portion control" is also known as "restriction." Essentially, when the stomach is smaller, you cannot put in as many calories. In Scopinaro's operation, the stomach held 40 percent of its original capacity, larger than the one-ounce restriction of the standard Roux-en-Y gastric bypass.

	Proximal RNY	Distal RNY	Duodenal Switch	Scopinaro's BPD
Stomach size	30 cc	30cc	120-180cc	250 cc
Common channel	500cm	100-400cm	100cm	50-100 cm
Common channel in inches	200 inches	40 to 160 inches	40 inches	20-40 inches
Biliopancreatic limb length in cm (not including duodenum)	100 cm or less than 15% of the distance between the Ligament of Trietz and the colon	For some insurance purposes, anything longer than 100 cm bypassed is considered a distal bypass	400 cm or about 60% of the distance between the ligament of Trietz and the colon	400 cm or about 60% of the distance between the ligament of Trietz and the colon

Bariatric surgeons have yet to determine the best relationship between the restrictive component of weight loss and the moderate "malabsorptive" component.

BPD Final Product

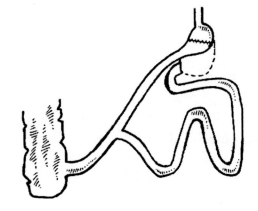

The Duodenal Switch

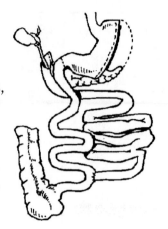

The duodenal switch is the most recent version of the biliopancreatic diversion. It is a complicated surgery, and in 2004 only about 40 surgeons in the United States are performing this surgery. This surgery is highly effective in keeping weight off patients, so some surgeons use this surgery for their patients who are considered super morbidly obese. However, some surgeons use this as their sole weight loss surgery option for patients, feeling that this is the most effective and long lasting of all weight loss surgeries. In addition to restricting the amount of food a person can eat, this surgery also has a "malabsorptive" component.

The Stomach

—to have, to hold, to chop

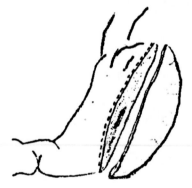

In duodenal switch surgery, about 80 to 90 percent of the stomach is removed. Part of the stomach is gone, not left in your body— but gone. Instead of your stomach looking like a canvass wine jug, it looks more like a long tube. The normal stomach can hold about 50 ounces, or 1.5 liters. After the duodenal switch surgery, your stomach can hold about 4 to 8 ounces, or 0.12 to 0.24 liters. This enforces portion control. Over time your stomach will enlarge a bit to accommodate a small to medium-sized meal (not a super-sized meal).

In the Roux-en-Y gastric bypass surgery, the stomach pouch holds one ounce, but the stoma is always open, so patients who have the gastric bypass can drink a lot of fluids. One of the keys to successful weight loss after the duodenal switch is a muscle called the pylorus at the end of the stomach. The pylorus is technically a muscular sphincter (as in, "yours is tight"), or a valve. It stays shut while food and fluid are in the stomach, allowing the stomach to work as a hopper and digest food. When the food is ready to go into the small bowel, the pylorus opens and the partially digested food enters the duodenum. Fluids empty much faster than solids. Because of the pylorus, food stays in the stomach until it is ready to hit the intestine, Technically speaking, the digestion allows the food to become iso-osmolar (did you really want to know that?). Keeping food in the stomach until it is digested prevents dumping, as in "eat it now, take a dump immediately after." Some consider dumping to be a key component of the RNY gastric bypass. However, there is no relation between dumping and weight loss and dumping is NOT fun.

Duodenal switch patients cannot drink a lot because the stomach fills and stays full until the pylorus opens and allows the fluid to flow out. Early in the post-operative period, if patients start to vomit, the area around pylorus swells and can keep the pylorus from opening and these patients may need to spend some time in the hospital getting intravenous fluids and not eating or drinking. The pylorus is key to weight loss because, unlike those with the RNY gastric bypass, DS patients can eat and drink at the same time. Remember, with the RNY gastric bypass, eating and drinking at the same time can push food through the stoma into the intestine, and you will continue to feel hungry. With the DS surgery, you will simply fill up faster if you eat and drink at the same time. This helps you to control weight later on as the stomach stretches a bit because, in addition to eating some protein, you can fill up by drinking a bit of water.

A healthy advantage to the DS is that you can add vegetables to your diet to help fill you up.

In the DS, most of the acid-secreting portion of the stomach is removed but the bit that is left can still cause an ulcer. Some patients will require life-long therapy with acid-suppressing drugs (Prevacid®, Pepcid®, etc.).

The advantage of this surgery is that if you develop an ulcer, your stomach can be completely examined with a scope, and sometimes the ulcer can be easily treated without surgery. Patients who have a duodenal switch can have aspirin,

Motrin®, Naprosyn®, Vioxx®, and other non-steroidal anti-inflammatory medicines.

With the RNY gastric bypass surgery there is always concern that pills can become caught in the stoma. This is not a concern with the DS so you can continue to take pills no matter what size.

Bezoars are very uncommon with the duodenal switch so you can eat fibrous fruits and vegetables that make up a healthy diet. Sometimes, a year or two following surgery, your stomach stretches and you may find you are still hungry even after you have had your protein. A healthy advantage to the DS is that you can add vegetables to your diet to help fill you up.

Some surgeons advocate doing this surgery in two parts. In the first operation, part of the stomach is removed (partial gastrectomy). This can be done fairly safely and through a laparoscope. This restrictive component allows patients to lose a fair bit of weight and come back later for "the switch" portion of the operation. Patients who are candidates for this include those who have very high BMIs, have many medical problems, and those who are on medicines that might not be absorbed if they have the switch. In addition, some patients' anatomy will not safely allow the bowel to be brought up for an anastomosis to the duodenum. Some patients may never need to have the second portion of this surgery done, as they may lose enough weight with the restrictive portion alone.

One of my patients had a heart transplant twelve years before he saw me. He needed another heart, but his weight had climbed so high he was taken off the transplant list. He was taking anti-rejection medicine, which is absorbed in the small bowel, and because we didn't want him to reject his heart, we did the stomach portion first.

The Switch

In the switch, a Roux-en-Y limb is constructed, but instead of draining the contents of the stomach into the intestines, it goes into the first portion of the duodenum. Since the average length of the small bowel is around 650 cm, this means that 450 cm of small bowel is not seeing food. The 450 cm of small bowel (give or take a few centimeters) is called the biliopancreatic limb. The biliopancreatic limb isn't empty, but contains digestive enzymes, bile, and a few other things.

The last 100 cm is where most absorption takes place. Some surgeons vary the size of this common channel. Some make this about 75 cm, some make it 125 cm. In the early days of the operation, many surgeons made this common channel 75 cm, but that did not provide some patients with enough surface to adequately absorb protein. These patients had to be taken back to surgery to have this revised to a longer limb.

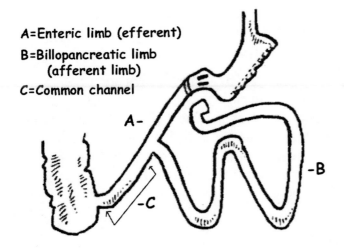

A=Enteric limb (efferent)

B=Biliopancreatic limb (afferent limb)

C=Common channel

Patients who are quite obese might be given a shorter common channel. There is no way of knowing if the limb will be too long or too short, but most surgeons are comfortable with 100 cm and most patients do well with that length.

The DS surgery can be done through a laparoscope, or an open or hand-assisted approach may be used. Hand-assisted laparoscopy is a combination approach, mostly laparoscopic, that allows the surgeon to reach inside the abdomen through a three-inch incision while also using a laparoscope.

Advantages of the Duodenal Switch

Several advantages to the duodenal switch surgery are:

- ability to use endoscopy to see the entire stomach
- no dumping
- ability to take non-steroidal anti-inflammatory drugs (aspirin, Motrin, etc)
- ability to eat fibrous fruits and vegetables

Controversies with the Duodenal Switch

Insurance companies may deny a patient payment for the duodenal switch in the mistaken belief that the malabsorptive portion is similar to the jejuno-ileal bypass. With the JI bypass, there were a number of long-term effects: the most severe was liver failure from cirrhosis. The DS procedure has been practiced since an article about it was first published in 1987, and it has been used for bariatric surgery since 1988. No long-term malabsorptive problems have been encountered with this surgery.

The forerunner to this surgery was Dr. Scopinaro's biliopancreatic diversion. He published his follow-up report of patients showing that his BPD was the most effective treatment of obesity. Dr. Hess, in Ohio, first combined the duodenal switch with the BPD, and his long-term results have also been published. Ultimately, many reports have shown that DS combined with BPD produces a more stable weight loss with fewer problems than BPD alone.

Unfortunately, in spite of clinical data that shows superiority of the DS over other procedures, it is still classified "experimental" by some insurance companies. None of the problems with the Jejuno-ileal bypass have ever been encountered with either the BPD or the DS/BPD. In fact, many of the problems encountered with the RNY, such as dumping, are avoided with the DS. The long-term data available for the DS is better than the data for RNY.

Some insurance companies have a hard time making up their minds regarding the DS, approving it one day, and then denying it another. Some companies may approve the DS in some states, and deny it by classifying it as "experimental" in others. Many patients have appealed this insurance company decision and the state insurance commissioner has overturned the ruling of "investigational" or "experimental" in a number of cases.

The best defense is to educate your insurance carrier about the long term results of DS and to show them the literature. Generally, patients go through a denial from the insurance company then have to appeal this decision. In the appeal, the medical director has some flexibility. While this is a lot of work, educating insurance companies is always helpful, not only to the person going through the process but also to future patients.

Not that I am cynical, but limiting access to medical care is one way the insurance companies save money.

Disadvantages of the DS

Some disadvantages of the DS are:

- patients tend to have loose stools – 3 a day average
- excessive carbohydrates or fats can lead to gas
- need for eating adequate protein to prevent deficiency

Because there is less small bowel available for digestion DS patients have an increased protein requirement (see Appendix One). Occasionally patients need prescriptions for pancreatic enzyme supplements to help them absorb more of the protein they are eating. This is an alternative to increasing the length of the common channel.

Laparoscopic Band	Duodenal Switch
Works by "portion control"	Works by portion control and also bypasses some intestine to limit absorption
Can be defeated with grazing, high-calorie liquids, and soft "mushy" carbohydrates	Can be defeated with grazing, high-calorie liquids, soft "mushy" carbohydrates
Works well with BMI 35-50 and is well suited for teenagers, women who wish to have children, high-risk individuals, and older patients.	Works well with any BMI. One of the few procedures that produces good results with BMI > 50.
Does not interfere with absorption of vitamins, but daily vitamins are recommended	Patients required to take multivitamins, iron, and calcium. Some may need B12.
Lowest rate of death and leaks, but revision rate is higher. Revisions can be done through the laparoscope.	Revision rate very low. Major surgical procedure.
Must chew food very well. No special requirements for protein.	All foods allowed. Protein requirements are 60-80 grams per day.
Foreign device is implanted	Stomach is removed and a distal bypass performed
Most common worldwide bariatric procedure. Approved in the United States in June 2001. Some insurance companies still do not cover this.	Most successful of all bariatric procedures. Some insurance companies do not cover the procedure.
Surgery time is 30-60 minutes. Hospital stay is typically 23 hours.	Surgery time is 2.5 hours or more. Hospital stay is 4-6 days.
Fast recovery and return to work in a few days. Requires follow-up and adjustments.	3-6 week recovery before return to work. Requires yearly labs.
No "dumping." Able to tolerate carbohydrates.	No dumping. Able to tolerate carbohydrates.

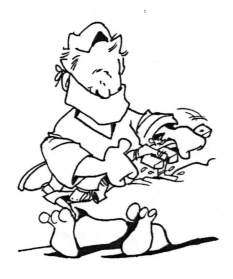

Ten

Surgical Revisions

Sometimes a patient develops a problem after weight loss surgery or a patient fails to lose weight, and his or her surgery is revised to a different type of surgery.

Some of the reasons for revisions are:

- unsatisfactory weight loss with a surgery
- technical problem with the weight loss surgery
- difficulties with the current anatomy (adhesions, pain, bile reflux)

The thought of a revision is probably a bit scary to those of you who are contemplating surgery for the first time. Those who had unsuccessful weight loss surgery probably want to hear more about it. The whole diet and exercise thing put you on a roller coaster that ended in failure. Considering surgery to revise a previous weight loss surgery can bring back guilt feelings. After all, who wants to be the only one on the block, or in the support group, to be stigmatized by "failing" weight loss surgery? There are many reasons for weight loss surgery failure that have nothing to do with you at all.

When a patient regains weight following weight loss surgery, a workup is done to find the reason the operation failed. There are two reasons for failure: anatomical and failure to comply. If the reason was anatomical, we can fix it. If, however, all the anatomy is normal but the patient has re-gained weight due to non-compliance, then revision to another type of surgery is unlikely to provide weight loss. The unwritten rule in weight loss surgery is that if someone has had two weight loss surgeries, both of which were "good" procedures with no obvious anatomical problem yet still does not lose weight, he or she is not a candidate for a third procedure.

Surgery for a revision has a higher incidence of all types of complications, from leaks to infections. This surgery is not to be taken lightly, nor is it to be considered routine by any means. There are some surgeons who specialize in revisions and have a great deal of experience with certain types of revisions. One of the best is my friend, Robert Rabkin in San Francisco, who has a great deal of experience revising procedures to a duodenal switch.

Valid reasons for revisions:

- Jejuno-ileal bypass (anyone who has this should have it taken down)
- opening between the upper and lower pouch
- stoma enlargement
- upper pouch enlargement
- recurrent stomal stenosis
- protein malnutrition

Jejuno-Ileal Bypass Revision

If you had a jejuno-ileal bypass surgery, The American Society for Bariatric Surgery recommends a revision. Their website, http://www.asbs.org, states: "As a consequence of all these complications, jejuno-ileal bypass is no longer a recommended bariatric surgical procedure. Indeed, the current recommendation for anyone who has undergone JIB and still has the operation intact, is to strongly consider having it taken down and converted to one of the gastric restrictive procedures." This should be done even if you are maintaining a normal weight.

The jejuno-ileal bypass was the most common weight loss surgery done in the 1970's. It produced dramatic weight loss, often 100 pounds in the first few months. There was no restrictive component of the procedure so patents could eat anything and still lose weight. Those patients who didn't change eating habits found that over a twenty-year period they regained their weight. But, that is not the reason that this surgery needs to be reversed.

There are several problems caused by the procedure. Calcium was not absorbed well because it complexed with oxalates and patients managed to get plenty of kidney stones and not enough strong bones. It is not good to have more calcium in your kidneys than in your back. Vitamin B12 deficiency was common because all but the last 35 centimeters of small bowel were bypassed, which lead to inadequate blood production, and thus anemia. Patients needed to have monthly shots of vitamin B12. However, the most deadly consequence was liver disease. The malabsorption combined with high caloric intake give patients non-alcoholic steatohepatitis (NASH). This led to liver cirrhosis and death from liver failure after the surgery.

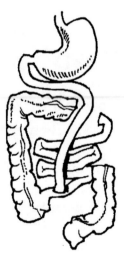

This operation has now been revised successfully to all types of weight loss surgery. The earliest revisions were to VBG.

Revisions from the Lap-band

Early experience in the United States indicated a high revision rate for the lap-band. Revisions were reported due to slipping of the band or problems that necessitated removal of the band. The lap-band is a device, and like all devices, at some point may fail. Balloons have broken and port sites have needed changes. The difference is that most lap-band revisions involve minimal laparoscopic surgery.

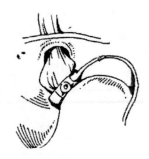

The band can erode into the stomach, but even this can be repaired through a laparoscope by surgeons who are experienced in laparoscopic procedures. However, some patients may require open surgery. Still, this surgery remains the safest of all weight loss surgeries.

Revisions from Horizontal Stapling

How to blow up a stomach

I live in the city that practically invented one of the first bariatric programs based on the horizontal stapling, so it is no wonder that this is the most common revision that we see at my hospital. This surgery worked well for a very short period of time. If the patient eats more than he should, the upper pouch easily enlarges to the original size of the stomach. This has to do with the anatomy of the stomach. The outer curve is greatly prone to stretch, and once it stretches, it keeps going. It is like blowing up a balloon. The first few breaths are difficult, but once it is stretched a bit it is a lot easier to blow it up more. The VBG was developed because the vertical staple line reinforced the otherwise thin portion of the stomach, making it difficult to enlarge the pouch.

This part of the stomach is thin and can stretch. As this pouch enlarges, it takes more food to fill up a person. Ultimately, the advantage of the "stomach stapling" is lost. This is why the "horizontal" stapling was replaced with the vertical banded gastroplasty.

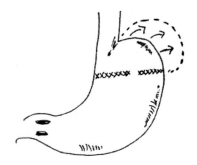

Roux-en-Y Gastric Bypass Revisions

The most common RNY revision is done when the stomach was originally stapled into two sections instead of cut (transected). A leak between the upper and the lower stomach makes the patient feel as if they can eat almost anything, and often they can. To solve this, the patient's stomach is transected.

The second reason for RNY revisions has to do with the pouch size. If the pouch has enlarged, revision decreases it to a smaller pouch. While this sounds fairly simple, it can be a technically challenging procedure and the concern is always that the blood supply to the stomach might be compromised This can lead to an increased incidence of leaks.

Some very obese patients have had revisions from a proximal to a distal RNY bypass. Mary is one of my favorite patients. She has a smile as wide as Georgia and a "can do" attitude that is infectious. She weighed over 460 pounds when she had a RNY proximal bypass. She went to the gym and water aerobics four times a week and lost nearly 100 pounds. Then she reached a plateau and couldn't seem to lose any more. On her evaluation we found her pouch was a bit larger than it should be and recommended that we revise that, as well as her small bowel, to a long-limb RNY bypass. Since Mary often complained of constipation, I assured her that by revising to a longer limb bypass we would solve the constipation problem. Mary had the surgery and did great. Mary also goes to

TOPS (Take Off Pounds Sensibly). She came in third place for the most weight loss in a year in the State of Arizona. Mary also is no longer constipated.

The stoma between the stomach and the intestine can require a revision. Often this stoma can scar and become too narrow to admit food, and even sometimes liquid. This can be dilated during an endoscopic evaluation, often with a balloon dilator (a balloon is put through the narrow stoma and inflated to a specific size, much like balloon dilation of a blood vessel). Some gastroenterologists are not comfortable dilating these and will recommend surgery to revise the stoma. If you need dilation, it is helpful to go to a gastroenterologist who is familiar with bariatric surgery and who works with a surgeon on a regular basis.

The stoma may need revision and this often has to be done in the operating room. If a stoma becomes too large, food will pass too quickly into the intestine and you will lose the benefit of the stoma. Recently developed procedures might allow a less-invasive reduction in the stoma size. In this procedure, the stoma is injected with a solution to make it scar to a smaller size.

Duodenal Switch and BPD Revisions

The size of the common channel is about 100 cm for most procedures. In the early days, some surgeons made this channel about 75 cm long and some of those patients developed severe protein wasting. This required the patients to undergo a lengthening of the common channel to allow more absorption of protein. It is rare to have a common channel revised to a smaller length for weight loss. The stomach might be revised instead.

The most common revision for weight loss failure is reduction in the size of the stomach. If the stomach becomes too large following surgery patients will not lose as much weight as they should. Revising the stomach to a smaller size frequently allows the patient to get off a plateau and begin losing weight again.

There are two reasons for a DS revision. One is if the common channel has been made too short, leading to protein malnutrition. The other is if the stomach enlarges, allowing the patient to regain weight or fail to lose weight satisfactorily.

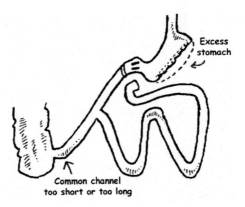

Excess stomach

Common channel too short or too long

Revisions from the VBG

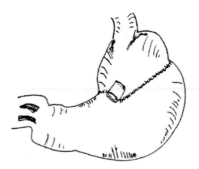

Patients who develop severe heartburn and a large upper pouch need revision. Generally the upper pouch becomes so large that it can block the stoma outlet, which only causes the upper pouch to become larger and cause more severe heartburn. Revision to a RNY cures this problem almost immediately. Revision of a VBG to RNY or DS is not difficult, and is often the next revision for those who were unable to lose weight with the VBG.

This Is Not a Walk In the Park

There are more complications with revision surgery than the original surgery. It takes longer, has more blood loss, and has a higher incidence of leaks, pulmonary embolism, and every other complication. These surgeries are not performed by every bariatric surgeon, and if your bariatric surgeon is uncomfortable with these operations and wishes you to go to another bariatric surgeon, please listen to him.

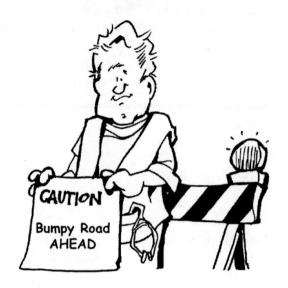

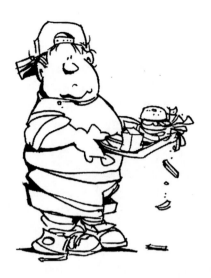

Eleven

Children and Obesity

I was lucky. Where I grew up the television didn't start broadcasting until 5 PM. There was no internet, and when we came home from school, our mom told us to go out and play. Now, our winters were a bit tough—I did grow up in Alaska. We had a lot of rain so sometimes we were banished to our room to play with our toys. But, when summer came, well, Mom let us out after breakfast, we came home for a quick bite, then back out the door we went. Yup, I remember those days—they were the last time I saw my ribs.

Now there is an epidemic of obesity in children. There are several obvious sources: the first is sedentary behaviors like me sitting in front of this computer. Television is now on multiple channels all day and all night. Internet has opened up even more reasons to sit for long periods. The world has become a tad more dangerous, and so moms don't like their kids going out all day. Keeping them in front of a television or computer screen seems safe. However, studies show how unsafe this is: they show that the more kids watch television, the higher their risk of obesity and diabetes.

The other difference between my childhood and that of children today is diet. There was very little fast food in Alaska—in fact, we didn't have any of the usual franchise operations. Our idea of fast food was putting peanut butter on some bread and running out the door to play hide and seek. Portions have also changed. Recently McDonald's had a sale of their hamburger for 19 cents so I bought one—my goodness is that thing small! It was the same burger they sold in the 1960's. Everything about that hamburger has increased: the calories, excess fat, refined sugar, and about the only thing that has not increased in size is the biceps on the kids who eat them.

As portion size in America increases, so does the gut size of our kids—and those of us who aren't kids, but that is for the rest of this book. Take a look at the traditional bagel you buy in any grocery store—it has about 70 calories. That is the one we used to eat. Now take a look at the ones in the Bagel Shop on the corner. These are larger bagels. Each one has about 350 calories—without the cream cheese. We now consume these at our desks with a large Latté full of cream and sugar as we sit in front of our computer.

Once upon a time, a child had two choices for school lunch: either he ate in the cafeteria, where the same government-regulated nutritionally-balanced meal was served to each child, or he brought his lunch from home. Two drinks were served: milk and water. Now the school lunchroom is like the food courts you find in big city malls. There are stalls where children shop for their favorite foods like pizza, hamburgers, and fries.

I remember when schools didn't serve desserts except on special occasions like holidays. Now there is an assortment of desserts and ice cream flavors to choose from. Students can also choose from a wide range of soft drinks during lunch and from vending machines between classes. (Remember raising your hand for permission to go get a drink of water from the fountain in the hall?) Now all a child needs to satisfy his craving for fat and sugar is some change in his pocket.

In the 1970's the average person consumed 27 gallons of soft drinks per year. The average person now consumes about 44 gallons a year. It adds up to an overall increase of 400 or more calories a day. There is not only an increase in the amount of sugar consumed, but also in the amount of refined flour. This is not just a problem in the United States, it is a problem worldwide. In Asia, where the diet is becoming more and more "American-ized," obese children are called "little fatties."

What can parents do to protect their child from a diet full of fat and sugar? We can't follow them to school and make their selections for them. The key is to start educating your child about nutrition at an early age. Serve healthy foods at home and talk to your child about what those fats and sugars do to a person's body. Point out the benefits of eating lots of fruits and vegetables. I wonder... what ever happened to "Popeye" the cartoon sailor man? When I was growing up we all knew "Popeye" was strong because he ate his spinach. I hated spin-ach but Mom explained that green beans and other green vegetables, if I ate them almost every day, would have the same benefits. Well, that didn't work, but then again I didn't want to grow up and go out with Olive Oil either.

Health-Related Risks

About 60 percent of overweight children have at least one heart disease risk factor by age ten, such as high cholesterol or high blood pressure. The health-related risks of obesity increase with time. The longer a child remains obese, the harder it is on his—or her—joints, on his heart, and the more likely he is to develop obesity-related disease such as diabetes. More "adult onset" diabetes, or Type II Diabetes, is being seen in adolescents than ever before.

The physical toll on kids is obvious, but the sad thing is that obese kids also have a lower quality of life. When a study was done looking at indicators of quality of life (QOL), researchers found that children and adolescents who are obese have a quality of life similar to those who are diagnosed with can-cer. Simply put, obesity in adolescents is devastating—not only because of the long-range health implications, but because of the low self-esteem that it causes.

Fatties

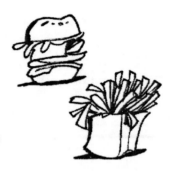

Children can be cruel, often without intending to be, when they call an obese child by nicknames like "chubby," "tubby," "fatty," or tease him about his size and weight. Parents can also unintentionally cause low self-esteem in a child by constantly pointing out to the child that he needs to eat less, or by comparing him to his "normal" siblings or to themselves, especially if the parents themselves don't have a weight problem.

The child's distress may not be obvious as he often covers it up with laughter and joking. The obese child often becomes the class clown in an effort to hide his unhappiness. Some, like Al Roker, turn this around and make this a positive effect, but they are the exception, and even Al Roker had to finally realize that health is important and has undergone gastric bypass surgery.

Exercise is the Key

The key to preventing early childhood obesity is physical activity. The Zuni Nation (a Native American group found in New Mexico) has instituted a program of physical activity, such as running, in their school system. This is early intervention to prevent diabetes when they become adults. The results have been spectacular. Physical education classes increase activity during school days, and there are more organized activities for after school programs. However, too often we see kids who are not enrolled in these programs hanging out at fast food outlets instead.

There are a growing number of "activity" camps for overweight adolescents. These camps have rigorous exercise programs and fun activities for children. They also serve healthy meals with proper portions, and in a gentle way, teach proper nutrition. There are also "boot camps" for kids, and a wide variety of other programs. While these are good for a summer, or a few weeks, the key to preventing childhood obesity is probably parent involvement in school and school activities. Preventing childhood obesity means developing good habits and following a program of activities all during the year, not just for a couple of weeks.

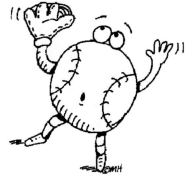

Motivating a child to exercise every day can be difficult. Some sports can be hard on an overweight child's knees, such as track, football, or basketball. You can't expect an overweight child to succeed at pole vaulting or the high jump. Insisting that a child participate in sports that he is neither interested in nor suited for physically is setting him up for failure, which further reduces his self-esteem. Swimming may be more his style and is gentler on the kid's joints. Dance is an excellent form of aerobic exercise for both boys and girls. The key to keeping the child in the exercise program is in finding one he enjoys. He may soon forget that it is an exercise program and begin to excel in the sport or activity. As he excels, he will begin to lose weight and gain self-esteem. Marathon television watching is not a sport, because if it were I would be an athlete.

When Diet and Exercise Don't Work

Now comes the controversy: should weight loss surgery be performed on children and teenagers? If so, at what age? Teenagers have clearly benefited from obesity surgery, but the long-term outlook is unknown. The same arguments that are made for adults are made for teens; that surgery is effective, and that diets and exercise, beyond a certain point, are not enough. The real question is, at what time, and at what level, do you go for surgery? A number of surgeons have lowered their age requirements for adolescents. Some have performed weight loss surgery on 12-year-olds, but most bariatric surgeons limit surgery to teens 16 years old or older. Again, as with adult patients, prior to entering a weight loss surgery program these patients must demonstrate that they have participated in attempts at weight loss through diet and exercise.

Some believe that lap-band surgery is well-suited to adolescents as it forces them to eat small portions, and it is quite reversible. Others will advocate that the duodenal switch is a better option as it allows one to eat a more normal diet. Still others will point to the RNY gastric bypass as the obvious choice since it has been studied for so many years. The pros and cons of which surgery is best for an adolescent probably will be debated for years, so let us start the debate here. There are chapters in this book about each of the major surgeries, but all the information related to weight loss surgery on kids is right here.

The Lap-band and Vertical Banded Gastroplasty

The lap-band and vertical banded gastroplasty are essentially the same operation, for all practical purposes. The major difference is that the lap-band is a bit easier to remove. Given the choice, lap-band wins out over the VBG hands down.

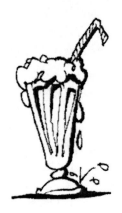

The advantage of the lap-band is that patients have no problem with absorption of any vitamin or mineral. The need for the adolescent to take supplementation is minimal. However, taking vitamins is the least of all the worries. Unfortunately, these operations can be overcome by the foods that all teenagers love—like milkshakes, chocolate, most candy bars, potato chips, or any high-carbohydrate food that has little bulk. French fries and other soft foods go through this pouch quite easily.

Some surgeons believe that a restrictive surgery will enforce portion control yet allow the adolescent, who is still developing, to grow normally without loss of "micro nutrients."

Roux-en-Y Gastric Bypass

Rou-en-Y gastric bypass has been used on patients as young as 12 years old by a number of surgeons. There is some malabsorption with this surgery, although if a proximal limb is used this is not an issue. The patient will still need to take vitamins and will need to be watched carefully by the pediatrician and the surgeon. The restrictive component of this operation can also be overcome with soft foods; however eating a diet high in carbohydrates may cause dumping with this operation. While there is no relationship between dumping and weight loss, the negative reinforcement might be considered quite cruel if the adolescent can never tolerate carbohydrates again.

The main issue with the RNY gastric bypass surgery is the inability to see the lower stomach, which is completely separated from the upper stomach. This is important because an ulcer can develop in the lower stomach. Under normal circumstances, if the patient develops an ulcer a stomach doctor, or gastroenterologist, can place an endoscope through the mouth and into the stomach and examine the stomach. After the RNY surgery, the stomach is divided in half, so the only way to reach the stomach is to go through the stoma and go around, but this is very difficult if not impossible to do. Other issues with the RNY surgery are that some surgeons do not like their patients to have foods containing fiber or fruits containing pulp. This can be a problem because fruit juices have a higher glycemic index than do the fruits themselves.

Roux-en-Y gastric bypass has been used on patients as young as 12 years old .

Duodenal Switch Surgery

Duodenal switch surgery has been used with several children who had compulsive eating disorders. DS allows a more normal diet: that is, one that allows fiber, fruit, and vegetables, and this is a plus. This operation also allows patients to have medications such as aspirin, Motrin®, or other non-steroidal anti-inflammatory drugs. The down side is that the DS bypasses a fair amount of small bowel. The concern over calcium intake in a patient who is still growing is a real one, as calcium is essential for growing bones. There is also a concern that a number of other "micro nutrients" which we don't know about yet might not be absorbed. However, this has yet to be the case.

It is essential that the surgeon who operates on adolescents have a close working relationship with the family and with the pediatrician. All of the operations work well for adolescents, and the right operation for the adolescent is going to be debated in the literature for a number of years. Taking vitamins and minerals, and careful monitoring of their blood levels is mandatory, as it is with adults. The possibility of needing life-long shots, or intravenous iron, or other supplements is real. A psychological evaluation is also essential and getting the counselor involved in the patient's care is helpful.

As with adults, these operations are life-altering. The child's life will never be the same again. It will probably be much better. Most children adapt well to the changes and look forward to being more like their friends and schoolmates.

The child's life will never be the same again.

The children love seeing the weight loss, they often feel better, and they participate more and more in sports and other physical activities. This should be encouraged and fostered. The risks of surgery in adolescents are similar to those found in adults. However, children seem to recover quickly from the operation. It's great to be young. It is fun to see these young people flower and enjoy their bodies.

When I was that age, I was fortunate. We had physical education classes that were intense and I lost a fair bit of weight during those adolescent years. Some kids are not so fortunate and some simply will not be able to lose weight without having surgery.

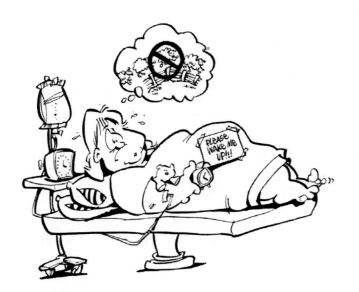

Twelve

Surgery: A Risky Business

When I give seminars to introduce patients to weight loss surgery, most patients come with their minds made up that this is what they are going to do. They have all done a bit of research and are anxious to have the surgery—and, in fact, want it quickly. I tell them right away that I am going to "scare the hell out of them."

Weight loss surgery is just that—it is surgery. The next three sections — *Risks of Surgery, Myths of Surgery,* and *Death of a Patient,* are not funny. There is nothing funny about surgery nor the problems that can occur. There are some simple things you can do to minimize risk, but all risks can never be entirely avoided. No matter how experienced or careful your surgeon is, bad things can happen. You may not heal well, your guts might leak, or you might have some underlying disease or serious side effects. So, be warned—this next section is the most important section of this book, so read it more than once.

You Will Wake Up

Your greatest fear is, "Will I wake up?"

Yes, you will wake up. I know this is your greatest fear. Every morning I face the fear that I will wake up and have to go to work. That's not the same thing? Okay. The risks of death while under anesthesia are around one in 10,000 patients. You will go to sleep, wake up and your surgery will be done. I love going into the recovery room and telling my patients, "It is all over, you are done, and you survived." It gets me a smile—or a request for more morphine.

The risks of surgery, any surgery, are real. The better prepared you are for the surgery, the fewer risks you face. This is an "elective" surgery, it is not an emergency, so if your doctor wants to put off this surgery in order to improve your odds, do it! Common reasons to put off surgery are infections, such as a cold, a urinary tract infection, or an impacted wisdom tooth. So if you develop a fever, get sick, or feel something in your body isn't quite right, call your surgeon. Putting off surgery for a week or two, or even a month, is better than spending extra time in the hospital with a problem you could have avoided.

Things That Can Go Wrong

Pulmonary Embolus

The main risk of death from weight loss surgery is the same as with every other abdominal surgery—pulmonary embolus (PE). This is a blood clot that breaks loose and travels from the legs or the pelvis to the lungs and lodges there, leaving that part of that lung unable to transfer oxygen to the blood.

This all starts from a blood clot known as a deep venous thrombosis (DVT). Most DVT happen during the operation when a patient is still, which can cause their blood to pool in the legs or the pelvis. Surgery tends to make blood coagulate more easily. This can be a good thing, but if it coagulates while in the blood vessel, it can develop into DVT. A classic triad, named after the famous Dr. Virchow, is called Virchow's triad. It states that DVT will occur when there is stasis, injury to the vessel, and hypercoagulability. Well, these two occur during every operation.

Surgery causes a hypercoagulable state—that is, a state where blood tends to clot more. Some medical conditions can make a patients' blood tend to clot. These include Leiden's disease, low levels of protein C or protein S, and some other conditions.

Surgeons do two things that greatly decrease the risk of DVT. First, they give you an injection of either heparin or a low-molecular weight heparin to keep the blood a bit on the "thin" side. If it is too thin it won't clot, and during surgery we want your blood to clot some. You will also wear sequential compression stockings on your legs. These stockings have little air activated pumps that pump up the stockings like a roller. You will probably wear these stockings after surgery while you are resting. These stockings work in two ways. The first is obvious—they keep the blood from pooling. However, they also work to keep the blood a bit thin.

The operating room is the most common place that these clots happen. The second most common place is after surgery while the patient is recovering. What can be done about that? Well, blood thinners help, but this is where you can help yourself—a lot. WALK. Walk, walk, walk, walk, and when you are done walking, walk some more. The more you walk, the less likely that the blood will pool in your legs or your pelvis. Walking has a lot of other benefits: you will feel better, you will recover faster, your body, especially your guts, will wake up sooner. I always tell my patients that I expect them to walk from the recovery room to their hospital room (in our hospital that is usually from the 2nd floor to the 7th floor). I haven't had anyone take me up on that offer yet.

The more you walk, the less likely the blood will pool in your legs or your pelvis.

As a preventative measure, a filter, or Inferior Vena Cava Filter (IVC filter), can be put in place prior to surgery to prevent blood clots from doing damage. This filter looks something like a birdie from a badminton game. This wire mesh sits in the main vein that returns blood to the heart and catches large clots before they can go to the lung. This, however, is not for everyone. As with all medical procedures, risk is involved with this procedure, so it is something you should talk about with your surgeon. Mainly, this procedure is used for patients who cannot be given certain drugs to thin their blood or those who have had pulmonary emboli in the past while on blood thinners. The filter is not 100 percent effective, and if a patient throws a lot of small clots, it probably won't help. However, for certain patients this is an appropriate measure.

Deep Venous Thrombosis

—or, blood clot in the leg

This happens to a number of patients and is the forerunner to a pulmonary embolus. If patients develop a blood clot, we place them on blood thinning medication for months and require them to wear thick stockings to prevent further problems. These blood clots can cause chronic leg swelling, painful legs, ulcerations and other nasty things. So, when your surgeon tells you to get up and walk, get up and walk!

Heart Attacks

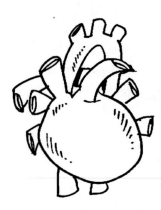
Some patients have heart disease, which in spite of the EKG or other tests, doesn't manifest itself until they have surgery. Heart attacks that happen after surgery carry a higher rate of death than those that happen outside of the operating room. So, if your surgeon wants you to have a stress test—don't stress, get it done! Remember, heart beats gut (paper over rock) and if they find you do have some heart disease, it is far better to get that taken care of before surgery than to have a heart attack during surgery.

Short-Term Complications

Other complications may not kill you but can be serious health risks.

Leaks

When a surgeon puts together bowel that has been drawn asunder, potential for a leak exists. An "anastomosis" is the term we use for when we put two pieces of bowel together.

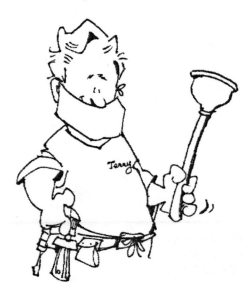

Just like when you repair a garden hose, if the two ends don't heal together well they can spring a leak. This often requires the surgeon to take the patient back to the operating room to fix the leak, or at least to drain the area. Sometimes patients spend weeks in intensive care, go to rehabilitation units, and have a prolonged course of treatment. Sometimes patients have drains in them for months before the leaks slowly close up. If you go back to the operating room you can count on, at the least, spending an extra few days in the hospital.

Anastomosis of any bowel can leak, they can leak for a variety of reasons, and repairing them doesn't mean that they will stay together. That is the frustrating part of surgery. No matter who does the surgery, how the surgery is done, or what sutures or staples are used, the connections between them are subject to variables that are beyond the surgeon's control. You might think that a surgeon can just open a patient up, put in a few sutures to sew up the leak, and everything will be fine—but it doesn't work that way.

Bowel is a living thing, and when you sew two pieces of bowel together a certain environment has to exist for the bowel to graft onto the other bowel and form a unit. Putting bowel together, or making an anastomosis, is a lot like grafting branches on a tree—the environment has to be correct for it to work.

When a patient has one leak, they are more likely to have another leak. So, even if the surgeon takes the patient back to the operating room and fixes them, the patient can leak again.

Well-meaning family members think this must be the surgeon's fault, but often it has nothing to do with the skill of the surgeon. The factors that caused the leak the first time may still be present to cause a leak again. Many things can cause leaks and inhibit healing. For example, certain chemotherapy drugs, steroids, radiation, cigarettes, infection, and some inflammatory diseases can inhibit healing. There are three main causes of a leak: the blood supply to the bowel can be a bit compromised so it doesn't heal together well, there can be some tension on the anastomosis that tends to pull it apart, or there is some mechanical reason for it not healing well. During surgery, many of us check the bowel for leaks, and while that eliminates one source of concern, we have little means of knowing how well the two ends will heal. Sometimes there are small leaks that seal themselves.

You can develop a leak days after the surgery, even though the surgeon took all precautions.

Bowel is put back together in two ways: some surgeons use mechanical staples, and some hand sew each anastomosis. Mechanical staples are engineered to a precision better than any human can sew by hand, and they are uniform and somewhat fool proof. The argument for hand sewing two ends of bowel together is that you can tailor it to the circumstances. It really boils down to preference. Again, your surgeon has a certain way he does things, so don't try to change how he operates because you like one way better than another.

Surgeons keep statistics on how many patients leak. Overall, if your surgery is done through the laparoscope, you have about a three percent chance of having a leak from the anastomosis. If your surgery is "open," then the leak rate is 1.5 percent. Again, each surgeon has his or her own statistics. Some surgeons have done thousands of surgeries with few leaks, so ask your surgeon about his statistics. This is one question your surgeon should be able to answer.

Patient, Heal Thyself

What you can do to prevent leaks

Suffice it to say, we are all very happy when patients heal well. There are a few things you can do to help yourself heal faster.

STOP SMOKING. Oh, did I make that clear? If you smoke, you decrease the chance of bowel healing together. People who smoke have tissues that heal poorly, as the nicotine inhibits the new blood vessel growth in the anastomosis. Smokers not only have a higher incidence of leaks, but also of hernias. So, if you smoke, stop. Some bariatric surgeons refuse to operate on patients who smoke.

DO NOT OVER EAT. There is certain strength to bowel and stomach—we call it "bursting strength," which is measured by how much pressure it takes to burst the bowel. When you cut bowel and you sew something new onto them, or you just divide them, the bowel is weakened. Over time the bowel regains a lot of its strength, but not right away. So, if you have a one-ounce pouch and decide you want to have an 8-ounce steak you might find yourself with a ruptured pouch and in a mess of trouble. Many surgeons won't let their patients have carbonated beverages after this surgery, fearing that the rapid expansion of the carbonation coming out of the liquid will cause a rupture or stretch the stomach or pouch. Drinking and eating at the same time is also hard on the stomach. Your stomach does not care if the volume it sees is from liquids or solids, and volume is volume. So for some weeks after surgery we don't recommend washing your food down with liquids.

What goes down well isn't necessarily good for you or your stomach.

WALK. The more you walk and get your body moving, the more oxygen and nutrients move around, the better you will feel and the faster you will heal—not only the anastomosis, but your whole body.

GET OFF THE NARCOTICS. We want patients to be comfortable, and we want them to be comfortable enough to walk, but we cannot take all the pain away. Narcotics slow the gut down. Patients feel bloated, uncomfortable, and constipated. The sooner you can get off the narcotics and get off the couch the faster you will heal. Plus, if your gut gets backed up you won't be able to eat well, your stomach stays filled, and if you eat anyway, you can over-fill it.

EAT PROPERLY. This seems obvious, but as your body heals it needs proper nutrients. You will not be able to eat much, and so some people eat what goes down well. What goes down well isn't necessarily good for you or your stomach. Mashed potatoes go down well but their nutrient value isn't as good as many other foods. We often have patients supplement their food with a daily vitamin. Bariatric patients need vitamin supplements more than anyone else.

If You Have a Leak

When a leak happens, particularly from the stomach, the acid from the stomach and some of the digestive enzymes leak out into the abdominal cavity and cause an intense burning sensation inside. This makes patients very sick, although sometimes obese patients don't show symptoms as quickly as non-obese patients. Early leaks are very difficult to detect.

The chemicals (acid and enzymes) from the stomach cause an intense reaction in the tissues. The tissues become swollen, and they don't hold stitches well. If you try to sew them, it is like sewing wet tissue paper together. Oftentimes they cannot hold a stitch and the only thing the surgeon can do is place a drain in the area and hope that the drain will carry away the noxious fluids, allowing the body to heal itself. Sometimes the surgeon has to cut out the inflamed tissues to find good tissue to sew, but often this isn't the time or place to do it. The drain will provide a place for the material to leave the stomach and the body will wall those materials off, protecting the rest of the abdominal cavity. If the body is unable to close off the hole, sometimes a surgeon can go in months later and repair it when all of the inflammation, swelling, and scar tissue has calmed down. Some leaks, however, when caught early, are simply sewn back together, and it just means a few extra days in the hospital. These patients are very lucky.

During this time, you need to good nutrition yet you don't need anything that might aggravate the leak. Your surgeon might insert a special feeding tube in your bowel or put you on intravenous nutrition (called Total Parentral Nutrition, TPN). You may need to be on this for months. Sometimes the insides become so inflamed and scarred that the surgery has to be revised. You might be able to have another weight loss surgery another time, but maybe not.

Can someone die from a leak? Oh yes. A leak is similar to a perforated ulcer. Once a patient develops a leak, he or she can become very sick and may require days or weeks on a machine to help them breathe. So, when the surgeon says you can go back to work in three weeks, remember—he means if everything goes well. In the best of surgical hands 1.5 percent of patients will develop a leak. Some of those patients will die, some of those patients will spend months in the hospital and rehabilitation, and a few lucky ones will only require another surgery.

Sometimes your insides become so inflamed and scarred that the surgery has to be revised.

What Is a Leak Test?

Surgeons always worry about leaks. We watch patients carefully for any sign that one might be developing so that we can treat the leak as soon as possible and prevent as much damage as possible.

Some surgeons, as a matter of routine, on a certain post-operative day, have patients swallow a liquid that tastes pretty bad. Then they order a series of x-rays that are designed to show if there is a leak. Some do this on the second to fifth day, but these tests are not always as sensitive as they might seem. Some surgeons check for leaks during the time of the surgery, and some surgeons do not. There is no right or wrong way to do this, nor does checking for a leak on the second post operative day mean that you won't develop a leak on the fifth post operative day. If a surgeon suspects a leak, then checking x-rays is an important tool. Some radiology equipment cannot handle patients who weigh over 500 pounds, so if you weigh over 500 pounds and your doctor suspects you have a leak, this is one test that your hospital may not be able to provide. We could just pump you full of air, submerge you in a bathtub and see if bubbles come out—like a bicycle inner tube. Just don't drink carbonated beverages before the test.

Leaks Between the Two Pouches

In the Roux-en-Y gastric bypass, some surgeons completely separate the upper pouch from the stomach. Other surgeons simply staple the stomach into two parts. If they are stapled, a leak might develop from the upper pouch to the lower pouch. This leak does not cause severe illness. Instead, it allows the lower pouch to fill with food, which results in patients being able to eventually eat more and more and lose the effect of surgery. Some of these types of leaks seal, and some do not. Some patients do fine with this, and others require surgical revision.

Splenic Injury

The spleen, a very vascular organ, sits next to the stomach. If the spleen is injured during surgery, sometimes it needs to be removed. Some quote splenic injury rate at two percent, although a study that looked at this carefully found upper abdominal surgery involving the junction of the stomach and esophagus (which is where we are) can have an injury rate of 11 percent.

The function of the spleen is debated so many surgeons try to save the spleen. However, sometimes it cannot be done with safety. The spleen is responsible for removing some items from the blood, especially certain forms of bacteria like the one that causes pneumonia. You can live very well without your spleen, but if your spleen is removed during surgery we recommend you have a vaccine for pneumococcus and one for meningitis if they are offered at your hospital. Typically, the vaccination should be at least six weeks after the spleen is removed.

Lower Pouch Distention

After Roux-en-Y gastric bypass, sometimes the lower pouch becomes filled with gas. If this happens it can require surgery, but sometimes a radiologist can put a tube in the lower stomach to keep it decompressed for a while. This can happen at any time to anyone who has had a Roux-en-Y gastric bypass, but typically it occurs in the first few weeks. Some surgeons place a feeding tube in the lower pouch, which can also serve as a valve to relieve the gas.

Wound Infections

There is always a risk of infection in the wound. We surgeons always worry about wound infections, but no matter what we do, they will happen to some patients. A wound infection typically happens about five to ten days after surgery. Usually the patient notices that the wound is getting red, the redness starts to spread a bit, and then some pus comes out of the wound.

Wound infections are easily treated. First, they need to drain. If the skin is closed over an infected wound it isn't allowed it to heal from the bottom up, the wound will "pus out" again. Second, you will need some antibiotics. You might also need to learn "wound care," like how to "dress" the wound. If you have a deep wound, it can take weeks and weeks to close, and can become a major nuisance. Sometimes the surgeon places drains in the wound or wicks, and sometimes special wound vacs are used. However, most wounds heal nicely when simply treated with some wound care and antibiotics.

Wound infections are typically caused by the patient's own bacteria.

Wound infections are typically caused by the patient's own bacteria. This is why we "prep" your abdomen with a special antibacterial solution before we cut into the skin. Various surgeons use different antibacterial preparations, and again this is a matter of choice. I use Duraprep™ because it kills most bacteria on contact and lasts for hours after the surgery is complete. This is also why surgeons give you antibiotics before cutting your skin. It is very rare that a wound infection is caused by the surgeon, some member of the surgical staff, or by "dirty" instruments.

After surgery, taking antibiotics will not prevent a wound infection but instead might make your body resistant to that antibiotic. That is why surgeons usually do not send patients home on antibiotics.

Bleeding

—or, "it was dry when we left"

Rarely do we have to take someone back to the operating room for bleeding internally. It does happen on occasion, and typically it is a small bleeder that opens up after we leave the operating room. After we finish any intra-abdominal surgery, we look around and make certain that the abdomen is "dry." A small bleeder can cause a major re-operation so we surgeons are careful to ensure that it is dry as dust inside the abdomen before closing the wound.

Internal bleeding can cause dramatic reactions in patients. Their heart rates rise and their blood pressure drops, and before we know it we are whisking them away to the operating room. When we open the abdomen we might find a lot of blood but sometimes we cannot find the source of the bleeding. This is frustrating but not uncommon.

Typical blood loss in surgery is anywhere from a cupful to more, so we expect the blood count to go down a bit after surgery. It will go down because of blood loss and it will also go down because, after surgery, we give patients a lot of intravenous fluid. Sometimes there is a lot of bleeding or a lot of bloody fluid draining from the abdomen. If you have this, please call your surgeon.

Abscess and Fluid Collections

An abscess is a pocket of pus, and pus needs to be drained. Developing an abscess in the abdomen means that something needs to be drained. Typically, these collections are drained in the radiology suite, which is great, because it means you don't have to go to surgery. Sometimes, unfortunately, these abscesses have to be drained in the operating room. There are a lot of reasons abscesses develop. It is a known complication of surgery. This will mean spending more time in the hospital, probably going home with the drain, and learning how to take care of it.

Evisceration

–or, "Hey doc, are these my guts?"

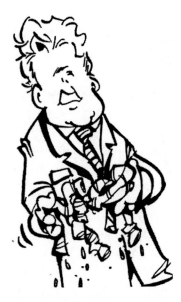

When we close the abdomen, we close the fascia, or gristle, with suture that is about as heavy as 30-pound test fishing line. Sometimes the suture is flawed and breaks, and sometimes a patient coughs or vomits so violently that the suture breaks. When this happens, the fascia opens and the contents of the abdomen, guts and all, bursts out. This is quite dramatic—because it breaks out through the skin and everything that was inside is now outside.

First, put your guts back inside of you, and then call the nurse. Second, if you are at home or there is no nurse nearby, put some warm salt water pads on your guts to keep them moist.

Then call your surgeon. He will take you back to the operating room and sew you up again. This rarely happens, but when it does it is frightening. It is also the cause of a lot of jokes, but it is only funny two weeks later when you are healed. If the fascia is torn or weakened and you don't have an evisceration, you can develop a hernia (see *Long term complications*).

Atelectasis

–or, "Don't forget to breathe"

Atelectasis is the most common post-operative problem. It is the source of fever during the first forty eight hours. When you have surgery you tend to take shallow breaths. Also, narcotics blunt your respiratory drive so your brain doesn't feel the need to breathe deeply. This can cause the small air sacs in your lungs to fill with fluid, and if your lungs become infected, then you develop pneumonia. Walking can prevent this problem, so walk the day of surgery and every day increase your walking—you will feel better and do better.

Long-Term Complications

Hernias

A hernia is a weakness in the fascia, or a hole in it, and stuff from the inside begins to find its way out. Fascia is the same thing as gristle—that tough stuff you can't chew too well. The fascia, and not the muscle, is what we sew together when we close an abdomen. When we sew you together we use suture, which is about a 30-pound test fishing line. When we sew the abdomen back together the fascia heals slowly: in fact it takes about six weeks for the fascia to be at about 60 percent of the strength it was before surgery. It can tear open, or rip (some people call it rupture) fairly easily. This is why we tell patients not to lift anything heavier than about fifteen pounds for the first six weeks after surgery.

This isn't a problem the first few weeks, because the incision is sore and will remind patients not to do anything too strenuous. But usually at about one month post-operative, people tend to forget and pick up junior. They sometimes feel a pop and then have a small bulge. The small bulge grows over time, becomes a bigger bulge, and at some point your surgeon will have to fix that hernia.

Hernias develop in about 20 percent of surgeries

Every surgeon has his favorite suture and method of closing the wound. Again—don't make your surgeon change what he or she does because you want it done a certain way. He is the expert, and if something works for him (or her), let him do his job.

Hernias develop in about 20 percent of surgeries, whether you have open surgery or laparoscopic surgery. Hernias need to be repaired. Hernia surgery isn't too much fun, but the newer techniques with mesh have made it an outpatient event. Some patients have a tummy tuck and their hernia repaired at the same time.

Adhesions and Bowel Obstructions

–or, kinking the garden hose

Adhesions are simply scar tissue inside the abdomen. After we do surgery, there is always formation of scar tissue. It is normal and natural. If, however, some bowel gets caught in the scar tissue, it can cause a bowel obstruction—which is like a kinking of the garden hose. This will lead to nausea and vomiting, you will stop passing gas from your rectum, and you will not have bowel movements. Or, you will blow up worse than road kill on a Jersey highway. This, fortunately, happens infrequently, but some people are more prone to adhesions than others. Surgeons can insert some material in the abdomen to reduce adhesions, but cannot totally prevent them. Some adhesions will also bind the bowel so that when you turn a certain way, you will wince a bit from the pain. While laparoscopic surgery causes fewer adhesions than open surgery, adhesions can still occur. A bowel obstruction typically occurs within the first year of surgery—but not always. One of my favorite patients was a little lady who had her appendix removed in 1905 in Kansas City. She came in with a bowel obstruction 80 years later, in 1990.

Stoma Ulcers and Strictures

In Roux-en-Y gastric bypass, the area where the small bowel is connected to the upper pouch can develop an ulcer or a stricture. The anastomosis can scar down to pinpoint, causing vomiting of all but some liquids. If this happens, the surgeon calls the friendly neighborhood gastroenterologist who will put a scope down and open up the stricture with a balloon. Typically it takes two to four sessions to open these strictures up.

Sometimes these are caused by an ulcer that develops at the anastomosis. This is one of the reasons we ask patients to always take some acid-reducing agent, such as Pepcid® or Prevacid®. Usually you will need to take this for life.

Gallstones

Twenty-five percent of patients develop gallstones during the weight loss, which is why some surgeons remove the gallbladder as a matter of routine. Some surgeons remove the gallbladder only if it appears to be diseased. A medicine called Actigall® works to decrease that incidence of gallstones in post-operative patients. Again, if your surgeon does one thing or the other as a matter of routine, go with what he or she recommends: do not make him change to something he is not comfortable with.

Nutritional Nuisances

(For more information about diets and nutrition,, see Section Three, Chapter Four, "Post Op Diet")

Lactose-Intolerance

Some patients become lactose-intolerant following surgery. If you become lactose-intolerant, a glass of milk can cause severe cramping and diarrhea. Milk is usually the worst offender but many can tolerate cheese, yogurt, or cottage cheese. For some patients, this is temporary, and for others milk becomes off limits.

Gluten

Celiac disease is caused by an allergy to gluten. Gluten is a substance found in wheat, barley, and rye. It can be difficult to diagnose Celiac disease even though it causes multiple symptoms. Patients can suffer from diarrhea, weight loss, and nutritional deficiencies (making it difficult to determine from a lot of other things that post-operative patients develop). This is a disease that can be unmasked by the surgery.

Minor Food Intolerances

Red meat is difficult to digest the first month or two following any of these surgeries. Rare is easier than well done and much easier than fried. This is unfortunate, because red meat is such a good source of concentrated protein. However, it does allow you to try new sources of protein such as tuna, Escolar (two great fish), some soy products like Bocca Burgers®, and maybe a smoked salmon (how do they keep them lit?).

In our post-operative diet and menu section we cover this more fully. Suffice it to say that your tastes may change for a while, and so will your desire for food. This plays great mind tricks, and patients learn what it is to eat to live instead of live to eat.

Menstrual Irregularities

—or "the cycle"

It is not uncommon for women to have multiple periods in one month or no period for a while. Clearly if there is severe and heavy bleeding you should see your gynecologist. But, if your periods are a bit askew for a while, there is a reason. This has to do with the complex metabolism of female hormones and the loss of fat cells.

Vitamin and Mineral Deficiencies

Flintstones, meet the Flintstones...

The National Academy of Sciences recommends that all adults take vitamin supplementation daily. Patients who have had weight loss surgery absolutely need this. You won't be able to eat as much as before, so you will need to supplement what you eat with vitamins.

Vitamin deficiencies are not simple to fix. They are, however, simple to prevent. So, take these warnings seriously. If you have a severe deficiency of some vitamins you can develop severe problems including dementia, reopening of wounds, and hair loss. (See Appendix Two.) There are a lot of vitamin formulations on the market, and a lot of patients go for the simple chewable children's vitamin or a prenatal vitamin. Various companies offer vitamins that are "specially formulated" for the bariatric patient—yeah, right.

A vitamin is a vitamin is a vitamin. Some doctors will sell you "special formulas," and if you want to help that doctor put his or her kid through school, then buy them. Again—vitamins are easy to take, deficiencies are not as easy to treat. and your body will not really know if that vitamin C came from a rose hip or was manufactured in Kansas.

Weight Loss Surgery Myths

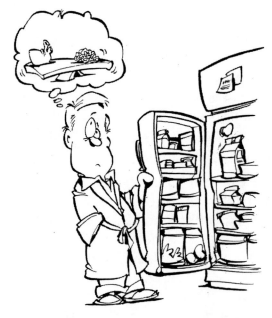

You can expect a lot of things from surgery, but there are a lot of things you cannot expect. So, let us go through a few of the myths that are popularized in the general press and find the facts.

MYTH: You can eat anything you want after surgery

FACT: Diet is a four-letter word and you will always be on one

Obesity is a life-long disease that requires life long treatment, and having surgery means that you will have to eat differently for the rest of your life. In fact, surgery means you will have to change your life entirely, and eat a certain way. Let me make this clear for you: **If you don't eat properly after surgery, you can die.** Surgery does not mean that you can eat whatever you want, whenever you want. This means you will be on a diet for the rest of your life. There are a couple of simple reasons for this.

First, you cannot eat as much. All weight loss surgeries reduce the capacity of the stomach. The average stomach is between 40 and 50 ounces, or about a liter and a-half. This means you can have a 16-ounce steak, a 12-ounce glass of water, the large basket of French fries, the nice spinach salad, and still have room for a glass or three of wine along with dessert. So this nice dinner at Morton's not only supplies you with enough calories for a few days, it also contains enough protein, fat, carbohydrate, and almost enough essential vitamins and nutrients to last through the first part of the week. By the way, I love Morton's. They even have a great chicken dish (Chicken Christopher). When your stomach is smaller, you cannot eat all of that. Practically, this is one reason we suggest that patients take vitamins. Since you don't have enough room to eat all the food required to keep you healthy, you must be careful that what you eat is going to sustain you. You need a certain amount of protein, carbohydrates, fats, calories, vitamins and minerals—if you do not get those you will become ill, very ill.

There is not one overweight healthy person who will trade places with a skinny sick person. So, you must learn about proper nutrition or at least develop a diet and menu plan that will allow you to sustain yourself. Fortunately, it is not that difficult to eat well, and if you normally eat well but just eat too much, then this surgery is a good choice to treat obesity. However, if you eat poorly you cannot expect your body to sustain itself with smaller quantities of food that has little nutritional value. In fact, you can expect that if you eat poorly, even if it is smaller quantities of food, you will suffer.

There is a condition where people crave certain things and this causes bizarre eating habits. One wonderful patient of mine was embarrassed when he told me that at night he would go outside and eat dirt from his garden. When we checked his laboratory work, we found that he had a deficiency in iron—his body was craving dirt because, as every Native Arizona person knows, we have a lot of iron in our soil. Once we replaced his iron, he lost the craving for dirt and his garden didn't get as much attention. Some patients do not receive enough nutrition through their diet. Even though they consume a lot of calories, they do not receive enough vitamins and minerals from their diet. You can super-size any meal, but if it doesn't contain the right stuff, you will feel full, but your body will still starve. Obesity is a disease that involves a lot of factors including genetic and environmental—one of the theories as to why some people consume so much more than others is their body is not receiving the essential nutrients they need, hence they crave more food. Just because you consume a lot of calories does not mean that you are nourished.

What happens if you do not follow through and eat well? You could die.

What happens if you do not follow through and eat well? You could die. You could experience simple, straightforward death, but it won't be a fun death—it will be slow and agonizing. You will have multiple organ failures, including failure of your liver and your kidneys. Before you die, you may become demented, you may become constantly tired, and you may have wasting of muscles and be unable to get out of bed.

MYTH: If you eat a good diet, you won't have to take vitamins

FACT: Your body may not be able to absorb enough nutrients to keep you healthy. Taking vitamins and supplements is easier than getting sick.

Prevention of vitamin deficiencies is easy and simple. You take a pill, or chew a pill, or swallow a liquid. Sometimes patients with weight loss surgery are required to take vitamin shots (I hate needles) and sometimes they have to take a lot of shots. In spite of that, *not* taking vitamins or calcium is foolish.

Taking Vitamin C Is Simple

Here is a simple one: You need Vitamin C to help with healing. Taking vitamin C is simple, and it is absorbed well and isn't toxic if you overdo it. Deficiency of vitamin C is a deadly problem, called scurvy. What happens is that old wounds open up. So imagine this: your abdominal wound starts to open up, as well as any other old wounds you have—not a pretty sight. It sure would have been easier to take the Vitamin C than to get your wound sewn up again. To cure scurvy you have to take Vitamin C, but you also have to get all of those wounds healed again, and that is not fun.

I choose Vitamin C as an example, not because it is something that people become deficient in, but it has such a great history. In the old days of the British Navy, the sailors went to sea for months at a time. If they were lost in the new world, and at sea, they had plenty of fish, which are pretty nutritious. What they didn't have was a source of Vitamin C, so these sailors became ill. Their teeth fell out, old war wounds opened up, and a number of them died. Then they discovered those sailors who had citrus fruits on board didn't get sick, so all British Navy vessels carried limes, and all sailors were required to eat a certain number of limes per week—hence, British sailors, to this day, are called "limies." And you thought you bought this book just to learn about weight loss.

It is amazing that such a simple thing could prevent such a horrible and painful illness. The same is true of weight loss surgery. You can prevent a problem a lot easier than treating a problem so please, take your vitamins. Perhaps we should call weight-loss patients "Vitaminees."

MYTH: Your surgery is done and so are your doctor visits

FACT: You have to follow up with your doctor (we like seeing you)

So you are doing what you should: eating well (which really isn't that difficult), taking your vitamins, and even going for walks. You are feeling good and loving life after having weight loss surgery. Do you need to see the doctor? Yes, it is very important, and you will need to have your blood drawn too.

I had this great patient, a very athletic guy who was over 500 pounds. He had the surgery, did well, but didn't come in to see me. He felt a bit winded, and had lost over 200 pounds when he decided to finally reply to my mail and make an appointment. This fellow was white. I mean, he was anemic as he could be. His blood count was about one-third of what it should have been because he was iron-deficient. We put him into the hospital and gave him six pints of blood before his blood count became just low instead of deadly. He had to have some painful iron shots after that. It took a while, but finally he started to feel better.

You Must See Your Doctor Regularly

Even if you have your surgery in another county, or state, or continent you need to see your doctor regularly. It does not have to be the surgeon; it can be your primary care doctor. At the end of this book is a list of blood tests that they should perform on you yearly. It is easier to prevent a problem than it is to treat one.

You should keep in contact with your surgeon. If they live far away, it might be difficult for you to see them, but have your family doctor send them test results, your weight, and let them know of any complications that you might have. Many surgeons participate in registries of patients, and for us to have accurate statistics, and long-term follow up, we need to know what is happening. Besides, we want to hear the good news and the bad. Finally, if we discover some new pill that works great with the surgery, or a better way to take a vitamin, or—God forbid, we find that the surgery needs to be reversed (as was the case in the jejuno-ileal bypass surgery), we need to contact you.

MYTH: All your health problems will vanish when you lose weight.

FACT: Skinny people get diseases too.

Strange as it might seem, skinny people get sick too. Yes, they do tend to live longer, but they still get sick. Skinny people develop diabetes, heart disease, high blood pressure, joint problems, sleep apnea, and a host of other problems. Just because you go from morbid obesity to a Slim Jim (or Jane) does not mean you are free of disease. Nor does it mean you won't develop the diseases that are commonly associated with obesity.

Orthopedic surgeons who need to replace a patient's knee or a hip refer them to me when the patient also needs to lose a hundred pounds. A good friend of mine was a general surgeon in Hawaii. He had a busy practice, and then his hips started to hurt. Eventually this thin, active man became debilitated and couldn't stand the pain. He needed both of his hips replaced. So, still in his 30's, John had both hips replaced and is now doing quite well. There are a lot of reasons that you may need to have the joints replaced besides being too heavy.

MYTH: You will not need to take medication any more

FACT: Skinny people need medicine to manage their diseases too

There are plenty of diabetic patients who are thin but still need insulin to regulate their blood sugar. Some have proposed that weight loss surgery will cure diabetes—it won't. While there are plenty of patients who have undergone weight loss surgery, and many require less insulin or go from insulin to pills, or use fewer pills, or even no pills—this does not mean you will be one of those. When you have diabetes, you will always have the tendency to have high blood sugar levels. While it is true that when you lose weight, insulin works better—it is not true that bariatric surgery will cure diabetes. You may still need shots or pills, and most certainly you will need to have a diet which contains a mid to low glycemic index.

Some patients need several medications to keep their blood pressure under control, and after weight loss surgery, while your heart may have a hundred fewer pounds to push blood through; you will probably still need high blood pressure medication. Thin people develop high blood pressure, and die of the complications of untreated high blood pressure. Franklin D. Roosevelt died of a stroke. His blood pressure was well over 200—and he was a rather thin fellow.

The Thin Person in Those Big Blue Jeans

Don't you love those before and after photographs? I don't. A lot of my patients have done great following weight loss surgery, but I try not to post their photographs. Somehow, I think of that as a bit of false advertising. Weight loss surgery can, by itself, only get you so far. Those patients who have gotten to a BMI of 20-25 did it with a lot of hard work, rigidly sticking to a diet, perhaps some exercise. We consider weight loss surgery a success if there is a decrease of 65 per cent of the excess body weight.

Ideally, we don't want to cut this too close (pun intended), and the surgery is designed to so that we don't. People who lose those extra thirty pounds really do it with help from the surgery, but they can't give surgery all the credit. Weight loss surgery, in whichever form, is a tool, not a solution to weight loss.

But, keep those old blue jeans; pictures of them make great post cards or Christmas cards for the relatives.

MYTH: Surgery is the easy way out

FACT: Surgery *is not* the easy way out

Surgery is not the easy way to achieve weight loss. You don't have the surgery and wake up thin nor do you become thin in a month or two. Surgery means you will have to live a different way than before. Surgery has risks, including death, and those who undergo surgery are putting their lives in the hands of someone else. Surgery provides a great tool for weight loss, it allows you to eat less and feel full. But there is nothing about surgery, nor the risks of surgery, that is easy.

MYTH: You can reverse surgery if you are not happy with the results

FACT: Surgery is not reversible

If you don't like a diet, or the diet doesn't agree with you, you can stop it. If you are taking a medicine for obesity, such as Xenical™, which inhibits absorption of fat, you can stop taking the pill (although some medicines have long-lasting effects). Once you have surgery, for all practical purposes, it is not reversible. Okay, sure, we can put bowel back together, we can make the stomach look the same, but it isn't like the original factory-installed equipment.

I once had a patient who had been told that her stomach stapling was reversible, that all the surgeon would have to do is remove the staples as they would from a piece of paper. But, that is not the case. You cannot simply remove staples, put bowel back together, and hope that everything will run the way it did before. Even the adjustable laparoscopic band (ALB) should not be considered reversible.

MYTH: Your life will be perfect after surgery

FACT: Success depends on your compliance and you may still have complaints

Anyone who has hung around the internet and researched weight loss surgery has come across the name of Sue Widemark. She has many different websites, including a website about weight loss surgery. People on Yahoo Group sites write about her in hushed tones, thinking that she is the anti-weight loss queen. She has quite a reputation, so imagine the day when I received an e-mail from her asking if she could attend my weight loss surgery seminar. She has her own Yahoo group, called WLS uncensored, that I now subscribe to. A number of individuals have had weight loss surgery and many of them have had very bad experiences.

It is difficult to determine who can and will comply.

Do these folks all have something in common? I asked. They did—most of them did not comply with their surgeon's instructions. Most didn't take vitamins or learn to eat well, or they didn't follow up with appropriate medical care.

One of my good friends, a bariatric surgeon in another state, had this very nice lady who came in for surgery. She had the surgery and unfortunately, afterward she developed a leak. She ate a lot of mashed potatoes, stopped taking her medicine, and didn't take her vitamins. She became ill and had to go back into a rehabilitation hospital. She had a complicated course of recovery then. When they measured her laboratory values, they found she was in a severe state of malnutrition. Ultimately, she had the surgery reversed (as best it could be). It is difficult to determine who can and will comply, but if you don't comply—you will regret it.

Now I ask all my patients to read and participate in Sue Widemark's website. It is (http://gastricbypass.netfirms.com).

Death of a Patient

The death of a patient is difficult for the surgeon, the staff, the family, and the support group. While this book is supposed to be a lighter look at weight loss surgery, the book would be incomplete if I didn't tell you that the ultimate risk of surgery is death. Instead of talking in vague terms, I will bringing you inside the death of a patient from my perspective. You do not have to read this chapter.

Helen was a wonderful person who wanted weight loss surgery so that she could get on with her life. Her life had been a difficult one: she was divorced and she had been estranged from her father for a number of years. Over the last year she had begun to make some positive changes in her life. She put aside her feelings and she and her father reconciled their differences. She also decided to do something for herself. She went through an intense weight-loss program and then came to me for weight loss surgery.

The surgery went well, and the evening of surgery Helen was doing laps around the nurse's station. The following day she was tolerating some liquids and visiting a few other patients in the hospital, offering them some encouragement. She advanced to some thicker liquids the next day and was proud when she passed a bit of gas. Saturday she wanted to go home, but since it was a bit of a drive, she decided to wait a day.

Sunday morning I received a call from the hospital. Helen was feeling short of breath and her oxygen saturations were declining. I told them to bolus her with some heparin (a blood-thinning agent) while I was on my way. They told me that her intravenous line had come out, and they couldn't start another one.

Driving the twelve miles to the hospital took no time on a Sunday morning, but it felt like an eternity. I arrived just as Helen was being placed into the Intensive Care Unit. I immediately placed a central line in her (which is a special line placed into the jugular vein) and we started the blood thinner. In spite of the blood thinner now coursing through her veins, she didn't get better. The lung specialist agreed that she probably had thrown a clot from her legs to her lungs.

Over the next 18 hours, I watched as Helen's life slipped away. I spent most of that time at her bedside, feeling helpless because there was nothing I could do. I talked to her father several times on the telephone and I knew that he knew she wasn't going to make it.

Helen had come to several of the monthly support group meetings and had made many friends. Although Helen was shy in public, the support group clicked with her and everyone loved her. When we announced on our website that she had died, many people responded with sympathy.

I felt numb. I have no idea how I drove from the hospital back to my house. My wife, a gastroenterologist (stomach doctor) reassured me there was nothing more I could have done, that I did everything possible. While I appreciated that, and my intellect knew that she was right, I still felt as if it was my fault. I really didn't want sympathy and couldn't be consoled. I simply wanted to go to sleep and when I woke up find that it was just a bad dream, but I couldn't sleep. That night my two dogs slept at my side. They knew something was wrong and wanted to protect me. They *were* protecting me—from my own demons.

A patient's death, for me, is personal.

The specialists who attended to Helen, the lung doctor, the heart doctor, the blood specialist, and her medical doctor, all reassured me that we had done everything possible, but I still didn't really believe them. Helen was alive when I met her, she had a great smile, and now she was gone. I told myself she really wanted this done. She had made the decision to have the surgery on her own. But I had done the surgery, and as a result her own body had killed her.

I went to my office and shut the door—something I never do. I put my head down on my desk and wondered why I had gone into a field where I was privileged to take care of people but cursed to see some of them die. My office manager came in and I told her that I did not want to do weight loss surgery anymore, that once I finished with my current patients, I was done. She knew enough not to say anything.

The support group was wonderful. Not only did they rally behind me and encourage me to come back to work, but patients of other bariatric surgeons in town emailed me and encouraged me to continue to perform weight loss surgery. The nurses at the hospital, in the ICU, and on the floor, were all wonderful. My hospital has a great weight loss program where a group of nurses are selected to work with these patients and given special training. Every one of these nurses came up to me and reassured me that they wanted me to continue to bring them patients, that these things happen. They encouraged me to "get back up on the horse."

A couple of days later I changed my mind about quitting surgery. A patient's death, for me, is personal. For my support group, it is personal. For the nurses, and the other physicians, it is also personal. However, it took my patients, and the patients of other bariatric surgeons to tell me what I already knew that the greatest thing I could do for Helen's memory was to keep working in this field, to keep doing weight loss surgery.

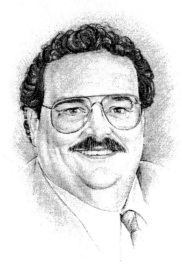

Bob

Bob was a friend of mine who died of pulmonary embolism. He traveled a lot, and airline trips are a risk factor for both DVT and PE. When traveling be sure to drink a lot of water and do a lot of walking.

Is It Worth It?

That is something that only you can decide. It is better to be overweight and healthy, than skinny and sick. But, an overwhelming number of patients who have weight loss surgery do well. Taking vitamins isn't that difficult. Seeing a doctor regularly isn't that difficult. Eating nutritious food isn't that difficult. This isn't like a diet that you can stop if you don't like it. Nor is it a phase. This is a life-changing operation.

Is it difficult to comply after surgery? After all, I couldn't stay on the XYZ diet plan?

Complying isn't that difficult. Afterward you will always be on a "diet," but it isn't something horrible, like having to eat a thousand grapefruits in a year, or eating only South African Zebra meat. It is fairly simple: eat the right things first, not dessert first; and remember, potato chips are not a meal. My favorite breakfast would be M & M's® (peanut, of course) with a glass of heavy cream—but I know that wouldn't be a good, nutritious breakfast. Learning to eat well is something all of us should do, and learning to eat less is something most of us cannot do without the aid of surgery.

It is difficult to stay on the Atkins diet forever. I love the Atkins diet, but I love pasta. With weight loss surgery, you can have pasta. Again, there are no bad foods, there are bad quantities of foods. After weight loss surgery you cannot eat the quantities you once did (well, some manage to do this, but we hope you won't make this your intent). So, this is what weight loss surgery isn't: it isn't a substitute for diet plans, it isn't something you can try, like a diet, and give it up if you don't like it. Every car needs a tune-up and oil change (okay, so I wrote this because my car hasn't had oil in 15 months—but hey, it is a patriotic act. I am saving oil so we don't have to import it). Every body needs vitamins, minerals, protein, some fat (not as much as we get) and some carbohydrates (not as much as we want). Everyone needs to see their doctor, and periodically get some blood drawn.

It isn't difficult to do, but it is important. Now, if you can do all this, you should have great results.

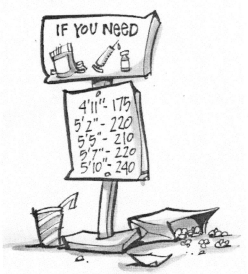

Thirteen

Insurance Company Woes

Do you think they are here for your health?

There is an increasing incidence of obesity in the United States and an increasing interest in weight loss surgery. Because of this, insurance companies are trying a variety of methods to limit the number of people who have the operation. Now, you are probably wondering why they would do this when the long-term benefit of the operation is so clear: decreasing requirements for various medicines, fewer long-term health problems, and so forth. However, insurance companies are bottom-line corporations. They care about what is going to happen this fiscal year, not what will happen in ten or twenty years.

Some insurance companies are that short-sighted. Imagine that you are an executive with an insurance company. Last year your company had to pay for a thousand weight loss surgeries. It is now March and you have already approved your first thousand payments. How do you decrease your payout?

Insurance companies use several tricks. First they require you to undergo several months, or sometimes up to a year, of a physician-supervised diet plan, so this puts off the surgery for a year. Of course, you don't improve, as there is no known diet plan that works well for morbidly obese people. So what do you do? Contact your family doctor and begin a physician-supervised weight loss program right away. Tell him or her that you want to come in to discuss your weight, meet with a nutritionist, and that you want to weigh in weekly. Tell your doctor that you need each weigh-in documented in your chart so that he/she can prepare a letter to the insurance company and outline your progress, or lack of it, and the need for the weight loss surgery.

Some physicians may prescribe prescription medicines and some may not—that is optional. Your physician may do some blood tests on you, check your cholesterol, blood sugar and a few other items before you begin. Having a physician-supervised program shows the insurance company that you are interested in your health and that you have tried to lose weight. The surgeon should not run this program and insurance companies will not accept such programs, so ask your primary care physician to start this process.

Another way insurance companies cut costs is by limiting the number of surgeons who specialize in weight loss surgery. In Phoenix, Arizona a lot of insurance company clients belong to health maintenance organizations (HMOs). Some HMOs now have only one or two bariatric surgeons do all of their work. Typically, this means that there may be only one surgeon in your area or HMO approved to do weight loss surgery. That surgeon may be quite overwhelmed and you might end up on a very long waiting list.

Garden State Leads the Way

A New Jersey state law requires that if the insurance policy covers the procedure and if the hospital is in the network, then the insurance company is obligated to pay the hospital bill (but not the surgeon) and the policyholder can choose the surgeon for the procedure. This means that you have to pay the surgeon directly for the surgery, which amounts to a little over $3,000. However, it is one way in which New Jersey patients have a choice of physicians that other states do not.

Policy Exclusions

Some insurance companies simply exclude weight loss surgery from the benefits offered. This is a devastating approach. Some of these exclusions are written very specifically and some are not. It is important to check the language of them carefully. For example, some insurance policies do not cover obesity, which is different from the definition of morbid obesity.

Remember that sometimes the best surgery for a co-morbidity of obesity is weight loss surgery. For example, while the insurance company might not cover surgery for weight loss, they might consider it for patients who need joint replacement, but the orthopedic surgeon will not replace the joint unless there is weight loss—so the surgery is actually for joint problems. Another is sleep apnea, which can be cured by weight loss. Therefore, while they might not cover surgery for weight loss, they might for the co-morbidity of obesity.

View policy exclusions carefully and if necessary, have them reviewed by a lawyer who specializes in this field—such as Walter Lindstrom at http://www.obesitylaw.com. If you don't understand the exclusion, if the exclusion is buried somewhere in the insurance policy or, if it is in small print, then you might be able to get this provision overturned. Mr. Lindstrom states that he has had success in overturning fifty percent of these exclusions. So, do not give up—do research and get professional help.

Famous Bad Insurance Company Decisions

Insurance companies have not yet realized how the World Wide Web has organized obese patients. One local insurance company made it easy for patients to obtain weight loss surgery and in the course of a year, many new policyholders switched to their company. They were shocked at how many came to their company simply to have their weight loss surgery covered. They quickly began to find ways to reduce the number of surgeries they would have to pay for.

Here are some of the more egregious attempts by insurance companies to keep you from having surgery. They:

- increased the requirement to a BMI of 50

- required you to sign up for year-long weight loss plan supervised by a physician

- gave exclusive contracts to one or two bariatric surgeons to limit access

- determined some surgeries are "experimental" or "investigational" (usually DS, long-limb RNYs and lap-band)

- approved lap-band but made patient responsible for the price of the band ($3,000)

- contracted with surgeons to pay less per case if they do surgery on more than five policy holders per month

Pending Appeal

Some insurance companies are truly interested in their patients' best interest. Recently I had a patient who decided the duodenal switch was appropriate for him even though his insurance company had a policy exclusion for DS. While appealing the case, he compiled a huge body of information about the DS and put it together in a binder. One of the medical directors of the company called me and said he was taking a leave of absence just to study the information so that he could bring a recommendation back to the medical policy board. That is a good insurance company (name withheld pending appeal).

There are many levels in insurance companies and some care about the health of their policyholders. However, insurance is a business, and with the rise of obesity and weight loss surgery, there will be more hoops to jump through as time goes on.

Why Not Pay Cash?

Some people wish to save up their money and pay for their hospitalization and fees with cash. There is one problem with paying for the surgery. Unless you live in New Jersey, you may not be eligible for any further care related to the weight loss surgery without paying additional fees. Still, if saving up money and paying cash is the only option you have, this can be the best investment you ever make.

Your Weight Loss History

If diets worked you wouldn't be reading this

One day a rather large biker came into my office. He was six feet tall and weighed over four hundred pounds. He had never been on a diet in his life. He had never even thought about weight loss until his bike needed some repair and another biker pointed out the dent he was making in his bike seat. When he came to see me, he didn't even know that surgery was an option. He had to wait for his surgery, however, until he had been on a physician-supervised diet for six months.

Surgery is a way of getting your inner biology to work for you.

Some people are super organized, save a copy of every diet they have ever been on—with physician supervision and without—and they know how many pounds they lost and how many they regained. Such individuals are rare. As difficult as it may be, put your diet history together. It will be helpful to your surgeons as they approach the insurance company.

Remember, your obesity is not a personal failure; it is not lack of willpower. It is simply a matter of your biology not working in your favor. Surgery is a way of getting your inner biology to work for you.

Results Not Typical

Disclaimer underneath most weight loss advertisements

About every fourth infomercial is about some diet or weight loss program showing a very attractive person who has lost 60, 80, or 100 pounds. However, look at the bottom of the screen. You will usually see "results not typical." My favorite involves one of my employees. Mary is a very attractive woman who had settled into a routine of eating out and cleaning her plate. A few extra pounds crept on; not enough to warrant surgery, just enough to be concerned, so she went into this rather expensive program. She lost the weight and the sponsors of the program liked her so much they used her for one of their commercials. One day I was sitting in the doctor's lounge, getting ready to do some weight loss surgery when I looked up at the television and saw my employee in this ad—now that was a bit of irony.

I always enjoy seeing those commercials. Usually you see a person jogging on a beach and telling the world how this drink, program, or device made them into the slim person they are now. Again, these results are not typical, but the commercials generate income from people hoping it will work for them.

Compliance

Compliance means that you, the patient, will do what your doctors asks you to do. If you do that, you have the optimal chance for success with the surgery. Compliance is almost impossible to measure pre-op. I ask patients to sign a contract with me. In it, they agree to come to support groups, stop smoking, and do a number of healthy things. Some insurance companies want an indication that a patient will be compliant following surgery, but this is, at best a guess. Ask any bariatric surgeon—we are surprised at how well some patients comply and how others buy donuts at the corner store on the way home from the hospital. There are always patients who will not be compliant even though they know the risk of harming themselves is staggering.

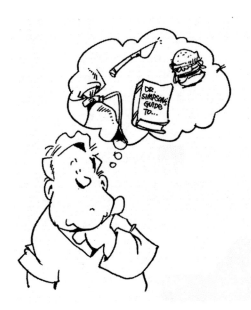

Fourteen

Which Surgeon and Surgery?

All the major weight loss surgeries work and all of them have advantages and disadvantages. If you select a surgeon first, then you will have the type of surgery that he is qualified to perform. If your community has several bariatric surgeons who do different types of surgeries, then you have a great choice. However, not having a choice isn't a bad thing either. Select a surgeon you can relate to, someone you have confidence in, and someone that can be your bariatric doctor for some time. Finding a surgeon is not like finding someone to work on your car. If, like most people, you have an uncomplicated surgery and recovery, then you may have little interaction with your surgeon. God forbid you should have a leak or some other problem, but if this happens you may have to stay in the hospital for weeks, then you may have to go to a rehabilitation center afterwards. If something goes wrong, then you want a doctor who is attentive, kind, and will help you through this process.

Don't insist on some type of surgery that the surgeon is not familiar with. If your surgeon's specialty is Vertical Banded Gastroplasty, but you read that a Roux-en-Y might have better results, don't ask your surgeon to change the type of surgery he does because of what you read. People are not all alike and you may not mesh with your surgeon. He or she doesn't have to be your best friend, but if you cannot tolerate your surgeon, then find another one. With some types of surgery, you may just want the doctor to do the work and forget about you. Bariatric surgery is not like that.

All of the modern surgeries have fantastic success stories, as well as horrific complications.

All of the modern bariatric approaches have their advocates and their detractors. All of the modern surgeries have fantastic success stories, as well as horrific complications. All surgeons have their complications, and if they have not had complications, well—they are better than this author. There is an old saying in surgery. *If you have not had complications, you have not done enough surgery.* Of course, a high rate of complications is not good.

Why Do Surgeons All Do It Differently?

Using the Internet to get advice

Often patients go to the Internet to find out what they should do. Our advice is simple: follow your surgeon's program. This is major surgery. Trust the experts. Your doctor knows you and he knows what he is doing, or he wouldn't be doing surgery very long. Using the internet to get a bit of advice is not only silly, it can be dangerous. There are a few things surgeons do differently. Here is a list of them, along with some of their reasons:

(a) **Abdominal binders for patients.** There is no evidence that a binder will prevent a hernia, but it will take the pressure off the incision until it heals better. Some surgeons worry that a binder will discourage patients from taking a deep breath, and thus contribute to lung problems. Some patients love their binder. It gives them a bit of security in the first post-operative weeks. Other patients find them cumbersome and don't like them at all. In either case, if your surgeon wants you to wear them, then do so.

(b) **Use of drains and feeding tubes.** Some surgeons use these as a matter of routine, and some do not. If you need to have a feeding tube, it is easy to put in during the surgery. After surgery it is harder to put in. The same can be said for a drain. Those who don't use them say the odds of needing them are small, and they can be placed later if needed. There is no right or wrong answer here, so do not ask your surgeon to change his way of doing things.

(c) **Leak tests.** Some use them before allowing patients to eat, some wait until there seems to be a problem. As mentioned previously—you may not have a leak one day, and the next day you may have one. Some surgeons feel very comfortable never ordering this test, and some surgeons order this test as a matter of routine before a patient leaves the hospital. Go with your surgeon's routine.

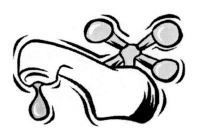

(d) **Use of various amounts of calcium and vitamins.** There are set values that can, and should, be followed. In the appendix of this book we have a list of tests that should be ordered and why. Often it is the internist, or primary care physician, who will order your test and follow these laboratory values. Too many supplements can be quite harmful and can be as bad as too little.

(e) **Post-operative diets.** Some surgeons like their patients on clear or full liquids for weeks. Liquids are much easier on a post-operative stomach than solids. Some surgeons advance the diet as quickly as the patient can tolerate it. Again, take your surgeon's advice.

(f) **Laparoscopic versus open procedures.** More and more surgeons are doing weight loss surgery through the laparoscope. This means smaller incisions, fewer adhesions (scar tissue) following surgery and less pain. However, some patients are not candidates for a laparoscopic procedures. Open procedures leave a larger scar but have a lower leak rate than laparoscopic. If your surgeon is comfortable doing laparoscopic procedures, and feels you are a candidate, great. If they don't feel you are a candidate, or if they start a surgery through the laparoscope and change it to an open procedure, trust your surgeon's judgment.

(g) The use of non-steroidal anti-inflammatory drugs, such as aspirin, Motrin®, and ibuprofen are okay to use with the duodenal switch. If an ulcer develops, a gastroenterologist can use an endoscope and possibly treat the ulcer. Some surgeons do not like their patients using these drugs.

(h) The common channel length is debated in the literature. Most have found that, for a DS, a 100 cm common channel is appropriate. At 75 cm there are a number of patients (5 percent) who will need revision because of protein malnutrition.

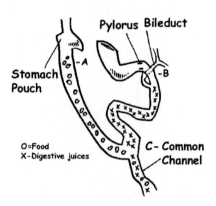

(i) The ideal length of the DS's enteric channel is also debated. Some surgeons will make it 40 per cent of the usual 600 cm of the small bowel, and others will make it 200 cm. There is no right or wrong answer, just a lot of speculation.

Ask Questions

Before you select a surgeon, ask some questions. How many surgeries has this surgeon done? Are you their first, their one-thousandth? Practice *usually* makes perfect, but not always. Some very busy weight loss surgeons claim that, because they do hundreds of these a year, they are good and careful surgeons and therefore you should trust them. There is something to numbers—the more you do something the better you are at doing it—most of the time.

However, this is not always the case. I was asked to evaluate a surgeon because he was in a bit of trouble with the medical board. He had a lot of experience doing a certain type of surgery, but it seemed like he was always getting in trouble. When I observed him performing surgery, I noticed he was a bit reckless and a bit rough, and I could see where he had a problem. We worked on a few things, I made some suggestions, and his results improved afterwards. By the way, he is now happily retired, which is probably best. The thing is, he had done far more surgeries than I ever had but practice had not improved his technique; practice had ingrained bad habits.

Technology often changes how we do surgery.

Some surgeons learn more with every surgery they perform. They try things a little differently here and there; try a new instrument or a new suture, or a new technique. They are always looking to improve what they are doing. When they find something that works, they stick with it. They are not afraid to try something new, but not afraid to do it the same way every time if it works for them.

Another measure is speed. How fast do they do the surgery? Well, speed can kill. I have seen a lot of fast surgeons, and when it comes to my body, I want someone who will take an extra bit of time and do it right. This isn't a race.

Before you choose a surgeon, check with medical boards, check with nurses, see if the surgeon belongs to American Society for Bariatric Surgery or if they are in the American College of Surgeons. The real issue is, do you like them? Do you get along with them? Do they have a program that you can feel good about? Do their programs make sense? So, how do you choose your surgeon? After you check several of them out, go with your gut feelings.

Before you choose a surgery procedure, a surgeon or a hospital, check these:

- Is the surgeon a Fellow of the American College of Surgeons
- Is he a member of the American Society for Bariatric Surgery
- Is the staff is friendly and professional – the staff often mirrors the surgeon
- Do the surgeon and staff communicate with you

Out-of-State/Out-of-Country Surgery

For a variety of reasons, patients may have to go out-of-state, or even out-of-country, to have their surgery. There are some fine bariatric surgeons in Spain, Mexico, Brazil, and other places that offer their surgeries for cash prices much lower than those in the United States. On the other hand, maybe you live in a state that does not have a bariatric surgeon, or your state doesn't offer the operation. Some surgeons and bariatric centers cater to out-of-state patients by offering a package that includes hotels, airlines, transportation with the hospital stay.

However, weight loss surgery is not like having your appendix removed. It requires long-term follow up. One reason for writing this book is to help primary care physicians understand what followup care patients need. Even if you have to fly or drive a couple of hours, make the commitment to return for checkups, and maintain contact with your primary care physician and your surgeon. Also, be aware that if you go out of town for your surgery, you may need to be hospitalized for longer than you anticipate, and this could be inconvenient for you and your family. Also, if you should suddenly have problems when you are at home, you may need immediate care and it may be impossible to return to your surgeon. If you are going out-of-town or out-of-state for your surgery, then first select a primary care physician who can keep watch over you, check your laboratory values and provide you with the support you need.

Bariatric Hospital, University or Community?

Weight loss surgery is an elective process, meaning that when and where the surgery is done is up to you, your insurance plan, and your physician.

Bariatric Hospitals

Bariatric hospitals are specialized places that only do bariatric surgery. The great thing about them is that they generally run with the precision of a Swiss watch. They are very organized and very friendly to bariatric patients—those wide seats are available. They have done this surgery a thousand times. It isn't something new, different, or weird. When you need an extra-wide seat, or a special operating room table, or a certain diet, it is there for you. Everyone at the hospital is there for weight loss surgery or because a relative is having the surgery, and everyone who works there is sensitive to your needs. You don't have to feel odd or different. Need transportation to the airport? It is arranged.

The downside is that if you have a complication you might need to be transferred to another facility. If you have a heart attack, there may be no cardiologist in the hospital so you might have to be transported to Our Lady of the Heart a few miles away. If you have a medical history of sleep apnea, you may need a pulmonologist who can arrange to set up your CPAP machine. If you should need an intensive care unit you will probably have to be transferred because most bariatric centers do not have one.

University Hospitals

University Hospitals are another extreme. These hospitals typically have departments for every specialty. If you run into a problem, a specialist is there to take care of it in five minutes. If you need an artery in your heart ballooned open, the cardiologist is there. If you have some strange skin reaction to the surgical prep used, the dermatologist will see you this afternoon. If you have to go back to surgery for a leak or you have several prolonged surgeries and now have a complicated wound to manage, the plastic surgeon is at your side to fix it up. If you have a complicated medical history with diseases so rare that your primary care doctor pulls down a textbook when you walk in the door, this is the place to be.

University hospitals have lots of people paying attention to you, and lots of people not paying attention to you. There is always a medical student, a resident, the attending surgeon, or some specialist to tend to your needs—but sometimes it is hard to get the nurses' attention. These are great places, but there is always the fear that you will be "experimented on" by the medical students or residents.

A teaching hospital is just that—where doctors learn to be surgeons, and they will be doing their learning on you. However, they will not be doing the surgery alone. I ran a training program at a medical center, and every stitch put in the patient was under my direction. In fact, one of my students did so well that he is now in charge of that same hospital! This does freak some people out a bit, but teaching hospitals provide superb care, they are on the leading edge of medicine, and they have the latest and greatest equipment.

Community Hospitals

Most bariatric programs are in community hospitals where you will interact with the surgeon who does your surgery. A lot of other surgeries are done there besides weight loss surgery. They are busy places. These hospitals may have other specialists in their facility, or they may not, it all depends on the size of the hospital. If the hospital has an ongoing commitment to bariatric surgery, then it has made the place friendly for the plus-size person's needs. Some hospitals have their own support groups and patients can attend these programs without charge.

How Hospitals Compare			
	Bariatric Hospital	**Community Hospital**	**University Center**
Organization	Set up well for bariatric patients and families	May or may not have developed a bariatric program	University Centers can have inefficiencies in patient care
Bariatric Friendly	Always	Variable	Variable
Availability of specialists	May be limited but may have transfer arrangements for patients with complications	Depending on the size of the hospital—can vary greatly	Excellent availability
Special equipment	Available	Generally available	Available

When choosing a hospital, look for the following:

- support groups
- wide availability of specialists
- if a smaller hospital, determine transfer arrangements
- availability of specialists if you have a specific medical condition
- commitment by the facility to bariatric patients
- radiology equipment that will support your weight

While all of these items are important in a bariatric program, all of them are rarely found in every facility.

I know of one center that has special arrangements for out-of-own patients. It sends a bariatric-friendly van to pick up the patient and family from the airport and takes them to a hotel. The hotel provides ample-size furniture and a special menu for the patients following surgery and for aftercare. The hospital picks the patients up from the hotel, brings them to its facility, and provides a shuttle service for the family. These are all very nice touches. However, the hospital stay is, hopefully, for only a few days. The key to this surgeon's successful practice is that he is available to his patients almost anytime they have a question.

Which Operation Should I Have?

If I am going to be cut, which should I choose?

Choices are a great thing; this is what America is all about. Most of your choices about surgery, however, are going to be made by your insurance carrier.

The Best News

You do have a choice! The downside of living in a society with abundant food stores is that we can store food all too efficiently in our fat cells. That storage unit can have severe and long-term consequences for your health. There is good news—we don't worry about famines. The best news is that weight loss surgery can give you a tool to take control of your life.

In weight loss surgery, we consider a 65 percent loss of excess body weight a success. What this means is that if you are 100 pounds overweight and lose 65 pounds, the surgery was a success. For all of you who lose more than 65 percent of your excess body weight, give yourself a pat on your back—the surgeon didn't do that, you did.

Calculate Your Excess Body Weight

Determine what your weight would be at a BMI (Body Mass Index) of 24 (see the all-famous BMI table). Your weight currently, minus the BMI weight, is your excess body weight. Now everyone who knows me knows that I am a nerd and I love math, and this stuff is great. Yup, I carry at least two pens in my pocket and I wear a pocket protector, but let's not get personal here. Here is a simple math problem with this that illustrates what I am talking about. If you are 5'8" tall, then a BMI of 24 means you should weigh 160 pounds. If you weigh 300 pounds (a BMI of 46) then you have 140 pounds to lose to get to your goal. If you lose 70 pounds in the first year after surgery, you have lost 50 percent of your excess body weight. If you lose 91 pounds, you have lost 65 percent of your excess body weight, and this is considered a success by weight loss surgeon's standards. If you lose more than 91 pounds, you have made it!

What Should Your Goal Be

But, Doctor I haven't seen that weight since I was 12 years old.

Every weight loss surgery patient needs a goal, something to strive for. Our goal in surgery is a loss of 65 percent of the excess body weight, but your goal should be much more than that. I always tell my patients to aim for a BMI between 19 and 24. It is like being a kid again. You can lose weight much easier than ever because you have a tool. Set your goal—you can make it!

Part 2

Surgery

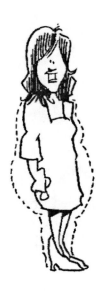

One

Approved!!!

There are several stages to weight loss surgery. The first stage is when you begin to think there might be a solution to obesity besides the endless cycle of diets. Then comes the research during which you learn all you can about surgery and its risks (and if you were smart, you purchased this book for that purpose). You may even know someone who has had the surgery. Then there is the price of the surgery. You worry that the insurance company will not pay for the process, and you worry about where you will get the money if they don't. Then you hear the next word—you are approved!

Suddenly you ask yourself—*What on earth have I done?* But there is no doubt. You made the decision to have your guts messed with and it is now going to happen. You fear the worst will happen so you will probably want to re-read the section about risks. Don't do that right away. Wait and enjoy the moment.

The next question is, "Can I do it tomorrow?" In fact, most patients ask me on their first visit to my office if they can have their surgery next week. I attribute this zeal to two things: the desire to get on with life in a new slimmer carcass, and wanting to get this operation over with before you change your mind.

So, now that you are going to the hospital, you might as well be prepared for it. Before you do, here are a few tips gathered from some of my patients:

A – Take a photograph of yourself, in fact take several. A lot of people don't like the idea of looking at themselves and have not had a photograph of themselves taken for years. This is the time to do it. When you weigh 40 or 50 pounds less than you do now, you can compare the before photograph with the new you in the mirror and feel good. Whenever you begin to wonder why you did this, you can take out the photograph and remember.

B – Measure yourself. Measure you neck, your chest, your arms, your waist, your hips, your thighs, your calves, your ankles. When you reach a plateau, and you will reach one, you will find that inches are coming off—and it is a good to watch them come off.

C – There are reasons you had this surgery. List them. If you have health concerns, such as diabetes, high blood pressure, or problems with joints, lists them. You can't expect those to go away immediately, but these health problems are made worse with obesity and they may improve now.

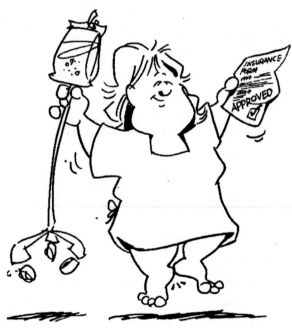

D – List the things you cannot do now but want to do. Some of my patients' favorite ones are to ride in a regular airline seat, dance with their spouse, tie their own shoes, and go into a store and buy clothes off the regular rack. If you want to dance at your granddaughter's wedding, write it down.

E – Start a walking program before surgery and if you cannot walk, then find a water aerobics program. You might be embarrassed because of your weight—don't be. Think about the people who will watch you slim down over time. These people will become your supporters. Start to get in shape now. You want to be in prime shape for your surgery.

F – If you have not learned about nutrition, this is the time to do it. Fortunately, you can find out a lot by reading this book. If your insurance will pay for you to see a nutritionist, then do so. Learn all you can about food choices and you will learn some interesting things, like how many calories are in a fast-food double burger with fries! The idea is not to feel bad about choices you used to make. The idea is to find some good choices for the immediate post-operative period and to learn more about the best food to eat in the future.

G – Go to some support group meetings. Talk to fellow patients. They will love to help you. Some of them will come visit you in the hospital. They know what you are going through, and—unlike your family (unless your family has frequent flyer miles with your surgeon) or friends—what you will go through in the future, and they will support you. Plus, they might have some protein mix for you or some clothes that might fit you. You never know. Just remember, a year from now you will have a chance to help someone and you will enjoy doing that. That should be one of the goals that you write down.

Now it is time to get ready for the hospital. There are a lot of things you can do to make your stay there comfortable as well as your arrival home easier.

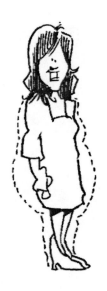

Two

Getting Ready to Go

Before you go to the hospital, go shopping. The last thing you will feel like doing when you get back from the hospital is stocking the refrigerator. If you insist on drinking petrified sawdust, try out the various protein drinks and shakes and find those that are least likely to ruin your taste buds. Many vitamin stores will let you sample a selection. Carnation® instant breakfast (sugar-free) is a very good choice. Sometimes it is not always in your grocery cases so you might have to special order it from Mr. Whipple (just don't squeeze the... never mind) your store manager. Likewise, Sustagen® pudding or certain drinks might or might not be available.

Don't overstock. Some people find their taste buds change after surgery and things you used to like may no longer taste good.

Stocking the Refrigerator

Some suggestions from my patients...

Sugar-Free Carnation®
   instant breakfast
Glucerna®
Sustagen® pudding
Ensure® pudding
Resource® diabetic drinks
Nutrimeal® drink
Isopure®
sugar-free popsicles
sugar-free instant Jell-O®
decafe tea
bottled water

sugar-free fudgesicles (see notes
   below)
clear broth (College Inn® comes
   highly recommended and
   there is a good assortment)
yogurt
cottage cheese
whatever protein bar you can
   tolerate
whatever protein shake that is
   approved
ice – either fresh or from the ice
   maker

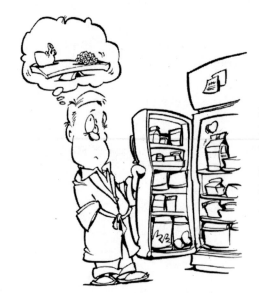

Some of my patients tell me sugar-free fudgesicles, are great for those "PMS moments." A water bottle with a sports top teaches you to really sip, instead of gulp, your water. Gulping water will hurt, no matter which surgery you have had, so learn to sip.

Several kitchen items will be quite helpful, so if you don't have them you might want to pick up the following:

- blender
- George Foreman™ grill (great for chicken breasts and other meats)
- popsicles molds
- shot glass
- Seal-a-meal™
- baby fork and spoons
- cup-size bowls

I don't expect you to be a chef, but some of these items will make your life after surgery quite easy. I am the last person to cook, honestly. My idea of preparing a meal is calling Daniel's for reservations. Baby forks and spoons are a great tool for RNY, VBG, and lap-band patients as they help you learn to eat smaller bites. Smaller plates and smaller portions is a great way to "see" a meal and not feel cheated. A cup-size bowl (no refills) is a great way to measure food.

Unstocking Your refrigerator

What is your Frankenstein?

You are thinking about stocking the refrigerator with items that you will need for the first few weeks after surgery, but what about all that stuff that is already in it, the stuff you used to eat? There are two ways to look at it. You don't need some of these Frankenstein foods nor do your family members, and not having them around for a few weeks won't hurt you. However, if other family members purchase and consume these foods, you will have to live with these. You will just have to develop willpower. If you purchased the candy for you alone and are the only one eating it—then you should consider getting rid of it. One of my patients drank somewhere between 12 and 20 cans of Pepsi® a day. After surgery, she stopped drinking it so she was able to lose 180 pounds and reach her goal weight. Months after surgery she asked her son for a sip of his Pepsi, and discovered she didn't like it at all. Sometimes your tastes change, and the foods you enjoy before surgery don't appeal to you anymore. That isn't a bad thing, especially if the food has no nutritional value. So, consider removing some of those foods from your house for a while.

Making the House Ready

—home, sweet home after surgery

Make the house ready for your convalescence before you have surgery. Here are a few items that will make life easier.

- Have grab bars installed in the shower
- Have grab bars installed by the toilet
- Get a hand-held showerhead
- Get a shower chair
- Stairs are generally not a problem if they were not before surgery, but make them safe
- Shop for some Medical Supplies for home
- Shop for at least two weeks supply of food or drink
- Modify your bed or get a recliner if you don't have one
- Buy a J-hook
- Stock up on baby wipes

Most people don't think about grab bars until they reach out for something to hold onto and there is nothing there. If you ever slip in the shower and grab for something, you will be glad you had them installed.

Several years ago, I decided to enclose the carport and turn it into a bedroom. The idea was for the bedroom to have its own shower, a separate entrance, and maybe a kitchenette. It really was designed with my folks, who are getting older, in mind. The shower was made extra wide to accommodate a wheelchair.

However, the grab bars were the key ingredient. Somehow, someone talked me out of installing grab bars by the toilet. Then one day when Mom was getting up, she grabbed the wall-installed sink. Yup, you guessed it. The sink came down. So, now we have a reinforced sink and grab bars.

A shower chair and hand-held shower head are great. A shower feels great after surgery, it won't hurt your wound, and keeping yourself clean reduces wound infections. A shower chair will allow you to sit down while you shower, especially those first few days. The hand-held shower is also good for getting to those hard to reach spots (the backside). Speaking of the backside, it is sometimes difficult to clean yourself back there, especially if you have an open surgery. A J-hook is a device made to hold toilet paper and extend your reach for wiping. The name pretty much describes how it looks. Some use salad tongs—and that might be the last use for those tongs, but there are some things your doctor doesn't want to know. Patients tell me that Martha Stewart salad tongs work best for this—honest, even I couldn't make this up.

A shower feels great after surgery, it won't hurt your wound, and keeping yourself clean reduces wound infections.

Baby wipes are cooling, flushable, and clean you up quite well, but sometimes you just have to get into the shower and use the hand-held showerhead to clean yourself up properly. I remember a great line from "Tuesday's with Morrie," where Morrie was slowly losing function because of a progressive neurological disease. Early on, he feared what would happen when his wife had to clean him. Later he said he learned that a true friend is someone who will clean your backside.

You will need to make modifications to your bed. It can be difficult getting in and out of bed following surgery. Some patients simply rent an electric recliner for a few weeks following surgery, other patients are fortunate enough to have a hospital bed. Most find that a recliner works well, especially an easy-glide or electric one. These things will make your trip home easier.

Stocking the Medicine Chest

You shouldn't need too much, but let me recommend a few things:

- Pepcid Complete®

- multi-vitamin—most people like some chewable form

- sterile 4 X 4 gauze pads

- hydrogen peroxide

- Tylenol®

- thermometer

- tape for your skin

- Milk of Magnesia® (for non-DS patients)

- glycerin suppositories (for non-DS patients)

Think of what you might need should the worst thing happen. If you have a wound infection, you might need to pack your wound with gauze a couple of times a day. Having some handy is helpful. If you have staples, you might find that putting a bit of gauze over the wound keeps the staples from becoming caught in your clothes. Gauze, paper tape, and peroxide are all things for your wound. Peroxide, by the way, is a great thing to clean blood and other body fluids out of clothes.

Pepcid Complete, a cross between Pepcid® and Tums®, is a great product to have on hand. It gives relief from stomach acid right away and also provides some long-term relief.

A thermometer is a great thing to have. Digital is fine. If you feel as if you have a fever, it is good to know your temperature. Most patients are what we call "bombproof" two weeks after surgery. They are beyond worrying about leaks or an abscess, not that these things don't happen, but they are so rare that after two weeks we usually breathe a small sigh of relief. Two weeks after her duodenal switch, Kathy called with a little bit of pain and a temperature of 103 degrees. She came back in the hospital; we drained her abscess and started her on some antibiotics. Knowing that her temperature was 103°F and not 100.3°F degrees gave her a "Do not pass Go, Go to the Hospital" card. She did fine (well, she might have a different take on it) but having the thermometer gave her the information we need to determine that she needed to be in the hospital. So, get a thermometer and use it. If your temperature goes above 101.5° F, call your surgeon.

Some surgeons give you prescriptions before you are admitted to the hospital. This way you can have your medicine chest stocked. Once you arrive home, it is one less thing to worry about. Many surgeons feel this is tempting fate and would rather write the prescriptions out and discuss them with you when you are ready to leave the hospital.

A few other things to do before you leave for the hospital:

- update your will

- get a living will

- establish a power of attorney

- pay your bills

- stock your refrigerator

- arrange for the care of dogs, cats, rats, fish, and maybe the kids

- make peace with your family, if you can

Make Peace with the Family

—but remember Bert and Ernie

I don't want to throw too much cold water on this experience, but before you undergo any major surgery there are three legal documents you should have updated:

1. your will, which states where anything you own will go.

2. a living will, which is your declaration of how you want to be treated should you need to be on life-sustaining equipment (please remember, there are many reasons to be on a respirator).

3. a power of attorney, which designates a person to handle your affairs, takes care of bills, and authorizes medical treatment should you need it. This is a bit morbid, but it can save your family a lot of headache.

Every hospital has stories of people kept alive against the advice of physicians because some relative wanted "everything possible done," even though there were "significant others" who knew the person desired to die with dignity should that time come. Such issues are hard to discuss, but do discuss them with someone you trust. Should that time come, a person who is armed with the medical power of attorney, as well as a living will, can execute your final wishes.

If you have a prolonged hospitalization, someone with a power of attorney can be sure your bills can be paid. Many companies have a clause in their agreement that if you become disabled, the payments to the credit card or mortgage are taken care of. Check those agreements out first.

I have a very soft spot in my heart for dogs. I cannot help it. I have two, Bert and Ernie, so patients with pets have my immediate ear. When someone tells me they want to go home from the hospital early because of their dog, it is impossible for me to keep them in the hospital. I am also fortunate to have a hospital where pets are allowed. There is never such a fine moment as seeing a dog and master reunited. So, make certain your pets are taken care of while you are away. It is also useful to check if your hospital will allow you to see your animal. However, I don't think too many hospitals will allow you to snuggle with your pet diamondback rattler.

What to Bring to the Hospital

- typed list of the medicines you take
- chapstick
- toothbrush
- hair brush
- robe
- loose fitting gym shorts
- open back non-slip slippers
- pictures of family and pets
- important phone numbers
- insurance card
- sweat pants and a top
- your CPAP machine
- reading or other glasses
- copy of your living will
- copy of your power of attorney
- fan (if you like sleeping with one)
- your favorite pillow and bankie

> **What not to bring to the hospital:**
> - cash and credit cards
> - computer
> - heavy reading material
> - any nice clothing
> - jewelry (including your wedding ring)
> - contacts

Getting ready to go to the hospital is both an exciting and a frightening time. The house is ready, the refrigerator and freezer are stocked, and your bills are taken care of. You have updated your will, your power of attorney, your living will, and kissed everyone that you can think of.

Usually the hospital stay is a short one, but there are things you can bring to make yourself more comfortable. First, bring some personal hygiene products. While the hospital can provide you with some of these, most people prefer to have their favorite toothbrush, hairbrush, razor, and other items. The air can become a bit dry at the hospital, so be certain that you have some Chapstick. Contact lenses can be more of a pain than not, so wear glasses instead. My female patients tell me that you might as well forget to bring a bra—which I have.

Every nurse will ask you what medicines you take, how often, and what allergies you have. So, type a list. Include the drug name, the strength of the drug, how many you take a day and when. In fact, make several copies of this list so the hospital has one and you have one. You have no idea how much time and aggravation this will save.

Modesty is a State of Mind, Butt...

Hospital gowns are rarely the right size. Our hospital is committed to the bariatric program and always orders the larger hospital gowns, but we find that once they are sent to the laundry we never see them again. I was on the obstetric ward (baby delivery) and saw one of our robes there. The mommy-to-be wearing it seemed to be enjoying it. For a bit of modesty it is always nice to have your own robe. Do not bring a robe that you care about; in fact, remember that this robe might become soiled with any number of body fluids, medicines, or who knows what. You might even consider taking a spare robe.

Modesty is not a high priority in the hospital, and the hospital gowns are designed so that we can get to parts of the patient's body quickly. We have to be able to get to the IV sites, the surgical wound, and any other site with ease. Anyone who has spent time in the hospital realizes that his or her rear end is probably going to be on public display.

I had knee surgery in the hospital where I was a surgical resident. Everyone in the hospital knew me, as I had been there since I was an intern, so when I came back from the operating room onto the floor I had a nice steady stream of visitors to wish me well. I had been placed in a machine that kept my knee slowly moving and was a bit groggy. The resident who was on the "pain" service had the same operation a few months earlier and told me not to worry, he would make certain that I had plenty of pain medicine. My brother stopped by and brought a six-pack of beer (more about this later). Between the Demerol and the beer, I was not feeling any pain from the surgery. Later that night, a nurse from another floor stopped by to visit and said, "Dr. Simpson, you're kind of hanging out there, let me fix that up for you." I learned that oftentimes in the hospital, you really don't care as much about modesty as you would normally. Maybe it was the painkillers, maybe the beer, but modesty was not a high priority with me at that time. However, visitors in the hall might not appreciate your disregard for modesty, so you might want to wear your own robe when you make laps around the nursing station.

Do not bring cash, checks, credit cards, or anything of value, including your jewelry. You don't need it, it can be stolen, and there are a lot safer places than your hospital room. You do need your insurance card and perhaps some form of identification. You will not need to write checks while in the hospital—write them out before you leave for home.

Some patients bring their cell phones to the hospital. This is not a good idea. Some hospitals expressly forbid cell phones (although my favorite hospitals are the T-mobile hotspot hospitals where you get great cell phone reception and have wireless internet service). Cell phones are easily stolen, and better left at home with a message saying you are out of touch for a few days (tell them there is no signal from where you will be as Edmund Hillary didn't leave a cell site there). In addition, there is some evidence that cell phones interfere with certain hospital equipment. There are always those who insist on bringing their cell phone and that is fine, Some hospitals don't have a problem with patients using their cell phones.

Heavy reading material, work from the office, your personal laptop computer—leave all of that at home. This time is about you and your recovery; it is not about anything else. This is your time. You will not have the energy, the ability to concentrate, or the desire to do the most mundane of tasks. Some people don't believe that. To say that Monica was driven would be a bit of an understatement. This lady strove for excellence in everything she did and decided the best way to become pregnant was to lose 140 pounds. She was a lawyer with a busy schedule, had a lot of clients, and she worked all the time, so she brought some legal briefs and her laptop (since we were a T-mobile hotspot hospital she had a fast internet connection). She never opened her laptop and didn't look at a brief, but she walked a lot. Monica is still driven but mostly now by her newborn son. Weight loss surgery is sometimes too wonderful for words.

A List of Your Medicines

–including any herbs or supplements

There are endless lists of what to bring to the hospital available to everyone, but one of the most important items is a list of any medication you are taking. Bring a list of *all* your medicines, including non-prescription vitamins and herbs. Make a note of the dosages and how often you take them. If your surgeon asked you to skip certain medicines before surgery, make a note of that.

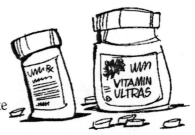

Also, note if you were instructed to take any medicines with a sip of water before surgery. You will be asked to stop some medications a week, or even a month before surgery. Some of these medications need to be regulated by other members of your medical team, and closely watched by them during the surgical experience. For example, Coumadin (also known as Warfarin) helps keep the blood a bit on the thin side (you will bleed easily). Some patients can stop this for a week before surgery without any problem at all, and some patients need to be converted onto another shorter-acting medicine before surgery.

Your physician may ask you to stop some medicines, such as hormones like Premarin, two weeks or a month before surgery because stopping them will reduce the risk of developing a blood clot. Your surgeon may ask you to stop other medicines you might not think about, such as aspirin, a week before surgery. All herbs and supplements should also be stopped before surgery, including Vitamin E.

The following table lists various medications and how they might affect surgery and surgical aftercare.

Drug	Potential Surgical Effect
Aspirin	Will decrease the ability of the body to clot. Should be stopped one week prior to surgery, or according to your surgeon's recommendations
Anti cholesterol drugs: Lescol, Lipitor, Pravachol	There is some evidence that people who have these might develop an increased problem with muscle breakdown during the operation. Stop one week before surgery.
Coumadin	Will decrease the ability to clot. Should be stopped four to seven days before surgery. This should be stopped only with extreme care by the physician who prescribes it for you.
Estrogen, Premarin, other hormone replacement therapies	Can increase the chance of developing a deep venous thrombosis and possibly pulmonary embolus. Should be stopped two to four weeks before surgery, under the care of your prescribing physician
Vitamin E	Can decrease the ability of the body to clot. Stop one week before surgery

Prevention Is Easier Than a Cure

It is easier to prevent a wound infection than it is to cure it. There are several things you can do before surgery to prevent an infection afterwards. Soap and water are the best preventatives against wound infections. Some surgeons want you to wash with special soaps, such as Hibicleans®, for several days before surgery. Hibicleans decreases the bacterial count on the skin, and every time you use it, the bacterial count is lowered even more. Some surgeons use Hibicleans as a prep solution before surgery.

Another popular product is Avagard®, made by 3M Company. This is an alcohol-based soap that quickly reduces the bacterial count on the skin, and it is combined with moisturizers, so the skin doesn't dry out so quickly. Both products work well, and if you can get them, by all means, use them before surgery. If you can't find them, use any antibacterial bath soap and water and keep your skin clean before surgery. This is a key to preventing wound infections after surgery.

To Shave or Not to Shave

–that is the question

Should a hairy man shave his belly before surgery?

No. If you are a hairy woman, still don't shave. Shaving can cause microscopic nicks in the skin that can become colonized with bacteria. Years ago, when we admitted patients the night before surgery, we had the nurses "shave and prep" the skin. When we stopped shaving the skin, we discovered that the wound infection rates went down. Now we shave patients on the operating room table or sometimes just before we take them to the operating room. We use a clipper on your belly so if you are hairy, don't worry, just use soap and water.

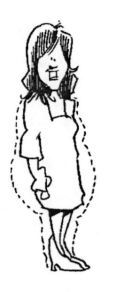

Three

The Hospital

Characters You Will Meet

Once you enter the hospital you will meet a full cast of characters. Each one plays an important role in your care before, during, and after your surgery.

The Lab Technicians

You will be asked to take a number of tests before surgery. These might include an electrocardiogram (EKG), chest x-ray, and some blood work. Your doctor usually orders these tests done a week before surgery so any abnormality can be checked out. However, one the day of surgery, you may need to have more tests. Some hospitals require you to have a blood test the week of surgery to check for anemia, and all hospitals require women who are fertile to have a pregnancy test the day of surgery. Even though you may feel you gave a lot of blood a week or two before surgery, you may be asked to give again.

Volunteers, Technicians, Nurses, the Sleep Man

When you arrive at the registration desk the first person you will probably meet will be a volunteer, although sometimes it might be a paid employee. At my hospital there are several people who fill this role. When I was a resident Mary, a Virginia Mason employee, was my absolute favorite. Mary was a friendly person who could talk to anyone about anything. She was smart, efficient, and knew where to have labs drawn or where get your x-ray done, and if the doctor forgot

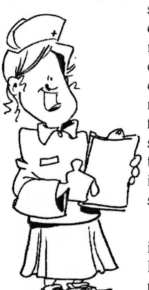

something, she would take care of it without batting an eye. When I needed my surgery done—I was a young resident then—she made certain any labs I needed were drawn (my cholesterol was checked just because I was curious). Mary, and her husband, John (honest, I am not changing names here, Mary and John) became good friends of mine. I knew them well (having scrubbed on surgeries for both of them) and have kept in touch with them all these years. They keep wondering when I am going to return to Seattle—and so do I, but that is another story.

Mary, or someone like her, will send you to the registration desk where you will begin filling out paperwork. If you were smart, you pre-registered, and much of this paperwork has already been filled out. You will be asked all sorts of questions, including history of drug allergies, allergies to latex, what medications you have taken, and, of course, they will want a copy of your insurance card. Once you have filled out the paperwork and they have verified your insurance (for the umpteenth time), someone will escort you to the lab to have some laboratory work done. If your lab work was done earlier, you will be taken to the pre-operative holding area.

The Pre-Op Area

So, who are all these people who make this system work? The first people you encounter on your way to the operating room are the nurses in the holding area. These "greeters" get you into the proper holy attire, start an intravenous line, and maybe even give you a little shave. If you need some blood drawn for the laboratory, an EKG done, or anything else, they arrange it.

Speaking of intravenous lines—or IVs—hey, these nurses are the best. They start IV after IV, day after day. Now, patients with obesity often are "hard sticks." That is, it is difficult to start an IV on them. Some patients insist that the anesthesiologist start their IV, but, trust me. These nurses start more IVs in a day than an anesthesiologist. Placing an IV is a skill. So relax, these nurses are pros—let them start your IV.

I had knee surgery many years ago, and my buddies, the anesthesiologists, decided to do me a favor and start my IV. Now, I have great veins—I mean I have pipes in my arms that you can drive a small truck through. After my buddy blew four veins, he went out to get another friend—cursing under his breath. I saw one of the pre-op nurses and asked her to start the line. She didn't realize that my buddy had already tried and in about sixty seconds, I was hooked up. My buddy was probably nervous about starting my IV, and the nurse just took care of me without regard for anything—she never did give me her phone number (oh, sorry).

Weight loss surgery is a team effort, and the anesthesiologist is a part of that team.

The anesthesiologist usually calls you the night before or the week before the surgery. Not all anesthesiologists do weight loss surgery Some anesthesiologists don't feel comfortable with heavy patients, but these are few and far between. I use a few anesthesiologists selectively, as do most surgeons. These are physicians who I trust to put my patients to sleep safely and who are familiar with bariatric patients. One hospital I visited was starting a weight loss surgery program and the anesthesiologists were upset. Many of them didn't want to work with these patients. The administration asked for my help with this. I asked if the surgeon who was coming usually worked with a certain anesthesiologist. He did, so I suggested they both come to the hospital. After several months, the local anesthesiologists began to change their mind and asked to be called for the weight loss surgery, but the surgeon remained true to his anesthesiologist. The moral of the story is that weight loss surgery is a team effort, and the anesthesiologist is a part of that team. Your anesthesiologist has probably taken care of many patients like you.

You will probably meet your anesthesiologist for the first time in the pre-operative area. Again, you will be answering more questions about medications, when you last ate, whether you wear dentures. Again, you will wonder if anyone bothered to read the chart. They did, but they need to hear this information from you. It wouldn't be the first time that charts got mixed up, two patients had the same name, or information was placed in one chart that belonged in another chart. They don't want to hear your entire history, just an abbreviated version of it. This not only helps them plan the anesthesia they will use, but helps determine if you need other medication while you sleep. If you have had anesthesia before, they will ask about your experience, whether you had a problem with anesthesia or became sick to your stomach after you woke up. They will talk to you about general anesthesia, maybe an epidural.

So, What Is This Anesthesia Stuff?

General anesthesia means you will go sleep. The anesthesiologist gives you some medicine through the intravenous line, you drift off to sleep, and then he puts a tube down your throat to help you breathe. During surgery, he will also give you a muscle relaxant so that the surgeon doesn't have to fight you.

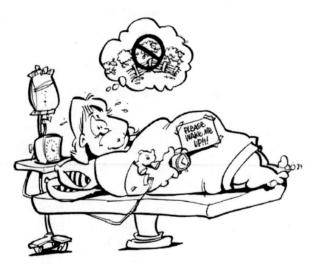

You will wake up!

When the surgeon is through with his work and you are all sewn up, the anesthesiologist lets the medicine wear off and you wake up. A good anesthesiologist has a "flight plan," or a "sleep plan," for the medications he or she will use during every step of the procedure.

Okay, so you heard the horror stories of people who wake up during anesthesia and can't move—oh, you didn't hear that one? Good. Ah, Dr. Simpson found another way to frighten his readers. Such events usually only happen under very special circumstances, typically during heart surgery or brain surgery.

The greatest fear of anesthesia is unfounded—that you won't wake up. Perhaps it is a control issue. For a period, your life is totally in the hands of a skilled anesthesiologist and a surgical team. During that time there are monitors checking every vital function you can imagine, from the quantity of anesthesia in your system, to your heart rate and blood pressure, to a catheter to see if you make pee. Of all the risks of surgery, not waking up isn't in the top 10,000. But, all humans, even anesthesiologists, worry about waking up—or rather, not waking up—after surgery.

Epidural Anesthesia and General Anesthesia

With Epidural anesthesia, a catheter is placed next to your spinal cord. Through this catheter, either local anesthetics, or narcotics, are placed to decrease your post-operative pain. This catheter is used after surgery too, to help decrease pain. There are some good things about epidural anesthesia—patients like it a lot—but not every anesthesiologist is skilled with it. If your anesthesiologist wishes to use an epidural technique, he or she will probably insert the catheter in you before you arrive in the operating room. Also, most of us who do this surgery use some agents to thin the blood a bit, and many anesthesiologists will not place an epidural catheter in you when you have these agents on board.

Many women have had epidurals during childbirth, and fathers who have been in the obstetrical area are thankful for its work. They are great tools, but they are not for everyone. Epidural anesthesia is rarely used for these operations without general anesthesia. There are a lot of reasons for it. You may be drowsy from the pain medication, but epidurals do not put you to sleep. General anesthesia really is needed for this operation, and you really do want to be asleep while someone like me is rearranging your guts. I had an epidural for my knee surgery—great stuff. You might want to be awake for knee surgery or to watch the birth of your baby, but do you really want to watch me rearrange your guts?

Once you are all set, wearing that stylish gown, donning the great blue hat, and ready to roll into the operating room, you will meet a couple of characters—although you may not remember them. They are the circulating nurse and the scrub technician.

The circulating nurses are a combination of go-fers and quarterbacks. They get items needed for the surgery as well as make certain that the room runs smoothly. If something happens, they are expected to pitch in quickly. Their job is a little like an airline pilot's—most of the time the job is a bit boring, but the take-offs and landings can be quite exciting. Before you go into the operating room, they will re-ask all the questions. They will ask if you understand the procedure you are having, they will check your name and make certain you are the person who is supposed to have this procedure. They will also check over your consent for surgery. If it doesn't say the right thing, they will call the surgeon to modify the consent, and ask you to initial or re-sign the consent. This seems like a terribly redundant step, but remember that people have gone into the operating room for one procedure and ended up getting another. They will again ask you about any allergies to medication, latex, to solutions used to prepare your skin such as iodine or alcohol, or to surgical tape or dressings. They will go over your medication list with you and again ask when you last took certain medications. They really do want to know when you ate your last meal, took medication, and a host of other things. They will check your blood type in case you need blood and will ask if you have a religious objection to receiving blood. They will also make certain that, if blood was ordered, it is present before your surgery starts. These nurses understand that you are a bit afraid. They will reassure you and make you feel better.

These nurses understand that you are a bit afraid. They will reassure you and make you feel better.

The scrub technician is the person who hands the instruments to the surgeon. You may not meet unless he helps you get from your hospital gurney to the operating room table, but these folks are critical to successful surgery. A good scrub technician is wonderful. When a surgeon and a good scrub tech have worked together for a while, the surgery unfolds like a fine ballet. As the surgeon puts his hand out for the next instrument, the scrub technician places it there. In surgery, we want things to go as routinely as possible. A good scrub technician anticipates and reacts quickly. I have worked with some scrub techs for years that I keep hoping will retire before I do. Others have my routine down pat after working with them only once. They are an important part of the team and if you have a good team, the surgery goes very smoothly.

The Operating Room

–into the temple you go

The operating room is where it all happens for the patient. It is here that the mystery happens, and this place is most frightening because the patient must totally give up control to the surgeon.

The operating room is a cross between the great temples of Delphi and the most modern NASA lab.

Like most holy temples, those who serve must change from their work clothes to special clothes. We must, before we perform the holy act of surgery, cleanse ourselves from the commonness of earth. The patient is taken from this earth into the netherworld; his or her very life forces are in the hands of someone else. While sleeping on the altar they are opened and sacrificed, they become different inside than before, and are marked with the holy scar. Now, the characters in the operating room—far from being priests in cotton pajamas, are more akin to a group of highly-specialized NASA scientists with randy senses of humor.

Operating rooms are filled with more technology than Microsoft can imagine, but we can rarely re-boot patients. In fact, if you go to a microchip factory, the employees look very much like operating room types because they learned sterile technique from us. If you look are looking for sophisticated backup systems and fail-safe mechanisms, your local operating room is the place to go.

I realize this doesn't sound very funny and it isn't. The operating room is a serious place where magic happens. It is where a patient is totally dependent on a team of people, their skills, their attention to detail, and for a period of time he is transported to the light.

During the operation, some surgeons like to play music. Some operating rooms have CD players that they give to patients and put the earphones on them, so during surgery they can hear their favorite music. Some surgeons love rock and roll, some classical, some pop. I am convinced, however, that most post-operative nausea comes from listening to country-western music. So, when asked what kind of music I like I say, "A.B.C.—anything but country." Some surgeons like the room quiet so they can concentrate. All have different styles and opinions as to how they want the room run. But make no mistake about it, when you are in the operating room it is the surgeon who sets the tone, determines the music (if any).

Recovery Room

Those aren't angels, they are nurses

You will wake up in the operating room but it is unlikely that you will remember waking up. However, you might remember being moved to your gurney from the operating room table.

Your first memory will be of the recovery room. Here is where you awaken from your anesthesia. I love seeing patients here and love telling them, "Hey the operation is over, and guess what? You woke up!" You will be in the recovery room for only a couple of hours. Here the nurses are trained to make certain you wake up adequately from your anesthesia. They will administer pain medicine so you are comfortable. They will try to balance the medication so you wake up yet are not in too much pain. They will monitor your vitals and once they feel you are ready, off you go to the next place.

The Intensive Care Unit (ICU)

Some patients go from the recovery room to the ICU. There are a number of reasons for this. For some patients who have certain medical conditions and may need one-on-one nursing, the ICU is a great place to be. Some patients with sleep apnea need to be monitored carefully after receiving a general anesthetic and narcotics. The narcotics, which relieve pain, also depress the body's urge to breathe—that is how an addict overdoses. Their body forgets to breathe. Patients with severe sleep apnea are sometimes routinely placed in an intensive care unit for the first day or more in order to monitor their breathing.

If a patient has had a rocky course in the operating room, the surgeon may wish to follow them carefully in the ICU for a day or so to determine if there is some underlying medical problem, or until they are stable. Some patients are given a lot of narcotics during surgery and simply do not wake up enough for the staff to remove the breathing tube. These patients are watched in the ICU until they are safely able to breathe on their own, or they are sedated overnight so that the tube can be removed in the morning. There are a number of reasons to be in an ICU, and it isn't a bad place to be. You receive very good attention from the nurses who are well-trained to take care of any medical problem that might arise.

There are disadvantages to an ICU—one is that the ICU is not designed to have patients walk. The other disadvantage is that they have very strict visiting hours, although that can be an advantage.

The Hospital Floor

This is not a spa

The hospital is NOT a spa. Sure, your insurance company pays far more for your hospital stay than a week at a five-star hotel would cost you, but this is a hospital. Like most hospitals, it doesn't resemble those on popular television shows.

In the past almost every hospital had a nursing program associated with it and there was a steady supply of good nurses available to help patients. Unfortunately, now there is a nationwide nursing shortage and because of this, there are fewer and fewer nurses who are available for patient care. As medicine became more complicated and nurses were required to do far more than pass medicines, take vital signs and make beds, the education of nurses went from hospital-based programs to university-based programs. This was one of the first steps that vastly limited the nurses available for floor duty. What does this mean? Once a nurse teaches a patient to get out of bed, it is the patient's responsibility to keep getting out of bed and not to wait for help unless they have some very specific needs. There are no nurses waiting around to help you do what you can do for yourself. Family members can, and should, help patients with some of their needs—but there are defined limits to this.

When you push the button for the nurses, do not expect them to be right there. Twenty minutes is the average amount of time for a nurse to respond to a call, longer in some hospitals, depending on how sick the other patients are.

Most patients will have a pump installed so that they can administer a narcotic for pain relief—called PCA for patient-controlled analgesia. This works very well and allows you to administer a specified dose of narcotic at frequent intervals. Do not let family members push this, only the patient should push this button. If you wake up, push the button and fall back asleep, only to wake up in pain again, you are probably doing fine. In fact, if you are sleeping a lot you should probably get out of bed and do some laps.

Family Members

-it is okay to love 'em and leave 'em

Family and friends can be of great assistance to a patient recovering from surgery. They can help the patient move out of the bed and encourage them to walk more around the hospital.

However, at nighttime I insist that family members leave the hospital and return to their homes or hotels to sleep. A patient's room is the last place I want family members to be sleeping. The reason is simple: a family member will get very little sleep in a hospital. The patient has 24-hour nursing care, something they will not have at home. It is important for family members to get some rest so they can help take care of the patient when he gets home—where there are no nurses to help. A number of years ago I did a fair bit of trauma surgery. One night a young lady was admitted after being in a car accident. She required some surgery to repair a liver injury. The surgery wasn't too complicated but the husband spent every waking hour at his wife's bed. Five days later I was on trauma call again and the husband became my patient. He fell asleep in his car and ran off the road. He was lucky; he just spent a very sore night in the hospital, but it could have been avoided.

Patients need sleep after surgery and when family members are there they get far less rest. Limit your visits to twenty minutes at a time, and if you plan on being at the hospital longer, go to the lounge and let your beloved sleep a bit. Finally, some patients are in more pain when a family member is present than when they are gone. We don't know why this is, but for some people it is absolutely true.

Family and friends are great support. They can assist you with getting out of bed, they can encourage you to walk, and they can even spot trouble before a nurse can. But remember, you will need them even more at home than in the hospital so, love 'em and leave 'em. Get your rest—your time is coming.

Day One After Surgery

Did you get the number of that Mac Truck?

The first post-operative day is usually the toughest. The day of surgery, you might take a few laps around the nurse's station, but mostly you will do a lot of sleeping. This is the day you will wonder why on earth you did this, or to quote about a thousand of my patients, "This is all going to be worth it, right?"

Different surgeons have different protocols for the first day after surgery, but no matter how you spend that first day, you will wonder what hit you. The good news is that by the end of the week that Mac truck will feel like a small Toyota pickup. I use that analogy a lot. One of my patients was hit by a Toyota— and she agreed with me.

Some surgeons order a swallow study to rule out any leaks from the surgery, and if that is clear, they will start to remove some of the tubes and allow you to begin drinking fluids. Other surgeons will start you on fluids from the first day. You will get through this and every day in the hospital will be a bit better. The best day is the one when some tubes start coming out.

To the Showers

A little soap and water will make you feel better

There is nothing wrong with taking a shower—in fact there is a lot *right* with it. Your wound can take a little soap and water about 48 hours after surgery, and your surgeon will no doubt want you up and moving. Your nurse may ask you to wrap up your intravenous line or do some other fancy stuff, but you should want a shower. There are a lot of great reasons to have a shower: (a) you will feel better (b) washing your skin will decrease the bacteria count and make a wound infection less likely (c) and, your roommate will like you more. DO NOT drink the water in the shower; your nurses need to keep count of all the fluids you take in by mouth, so don't fool them with this trick.

What Is This Stuff Painted On Me?

The prep solution we use for the abdomen is probably still lingering. I use DuraPrep®, which is fast-acting and kills a lot of the skin bacteria. This solution stays on the skin and kills bacteria for up to 12 hours. It can't be scrubbed off with soap and water but there is a product that will remove it. Some doctors use iodine solutions that come off easily with soap and water.

Again, your first shower should be a fun time where you simply let the water run over your abdomen. Enjoy looking at that belly, because you will see less of it as the days continue. I belong to a country club, and one day I was asked to come see the manager of the club. I was wondering what on earth I had done, when he asked if I would write a note for a member. Apparently, a member had surgery on his knee and the Betadyne® solution came off in the shower. Someone in the downstream area saw the iodine in the water and turned the fellow in for peeing in the shower (see, and you thought you bought this book just to learn about weight loss surgery). The fellow is still a member, and he didn't get a nasty letter from the club.

Taking Care of Your Wound

Every surgeon has a different way of closing the wound, and every wound is a bit different. Whether you had laparoscopic bypass or open, somewhere you have a little reminder that someone went inside of you and rearranged a few guts. The surgeon may have closed your skin with sutures that will dissolve, or he may have used a fibrin sealant (our version of superglue), or staples. There are a lot of ways to close a wound, but no matter which one your surgeon used, taking care of it is easy.

After 48 hours you can wash it with soap and water—in fact we want you to wash it. Pat the wound dry and allow air to come in contact with it. Do not put Neosporin®, or other ointments on it unless otherwise directed. If you have staples and they are catching on clothes, put a gauze over them.

The Incentive Spirometer

–suck, don't blow

Many surgeons or nurses will give you this cute little device that has a mouthpiece attached to a bubble. The deeper the breath you take, the higher the bubble goes. The idea of this is to encourage you to take slow, deep breaths. If you don't take slow, deep breaths your lungs will not become expanded, and they can fill up with fluid, causing you to run a fever. If the fluid becomes infected you can develop pneumonia, and the last thing you want is to have to cough with a fresh incision. If you don't get an incentive spirometer, ask for one. They are a great device and even before surgery, you can test yourself. This will give you a goal to reach after the operation. How often should you suck on this device? Anytime there is a commercial on television, suck it up. When patients first see the device they think that it is to blow in but that will do nothing except tire you out.

Walk, Walk Some More

Do the Olympic Nurse Station Triathlon

There is no secret to getting better in the hospital—the answer is simple — you walk. Walking will do a lot of things for you. First it will make you feel better. Second, it is the best thing that you can do to prevent pulmonary embolus—so when you don't feel like walking... Third, the more you walk the fewer drugs you will need. We don't know why this is, but the more a patient gets up and around the less they need pain killers, and the better they feel. Finally, your guts recover quicker.

I have heard every excuse to not walk after surgery, but I am sure there will be a few more invented. The nurse, or some staff member, will help you get up the first time, and after that it is up to you. How much and how far? Simple— you start walking and you stop when the nurses tell you that you are making them dizzy.

Every now and then there are exceptions to this, but the best way to get out of the hospital with as few problems as you can expect is to walk. Oh, the triathlon—one lap around the nurses station, followed by a shower, then some quality breaths with your incentive spirometer!

"Hey Doc, When Can I Go Home?"

Surgeons have their own protocols as to when you can leave the hospital. Some are more conservative than others. These are dependent upon several factors: first you have to be able to take in enough liquids so you won't become depleted; second, you have to be comfortable on oral pain medicine. Some surgeons like for you to pass some gas (flatus, not burps) before leaving, and others want you to have a bowel movement. There are other reasons also—one of my patients was ready to go home on Thursday but wanted to wait a day, so Friday morning I was pleased to start signing her discharge papers, as she was getting a bit anxious. A friend of mine called me and said, "Don't you understand, she wants to go home when her mom gets in town," (her mother was coming on Saturday). "Her husband probably won't do anything with the kids and this lady has to go home and do everything." She was right, so Samantha stayed an extra day until her mom arrived to take care of all the household chores. Sometimes even we doctors have to know more about patients than how well they are doing physically—or, as my friends from the east would tell me, "Doink!"

Laparoscopic patients, depending upon the procedure, surgeon's protocol, and a few other assorted things, can go home anywhere from the second post-operative day onward. Patients who have had "open" surgery can go home anywhere from the third post-operative day onward. Again, this is highly dependent upon what your surgeon wants you to do. If they want you to wait until you have passed a bit of gas, that is fine.

A Few Tubes–How to Care For Them

Every surgeon uses a different number of tubes that go in various body cavities. Some surgeons use every tube known to man, and some use very few of them.

Tube type	Use of the tube	When it is removed
Foley catheter	This tube is placed in the bladder of the patient and helps to monitor urine output.	Often removed the first or second day after surgery if urine output is steady
Nasogastric tube The NG	This tube goes from your nose into your stomach or pouch. It is used to decompress the stomach to avoid it from stretching too fast	Removed after a leak test confirms no leak. Some remove these the first to third day after surgery.
Drainage tubes Jackson-Pratt (JP) Blake Tube Hemovac Penrose drain	These are various types of drains that are placed in the abdomen. They can drain an abscess, a leak, bile, etc.	Removed anywhere from a few days to a week. If there is a leak these tubes remain in place until the body has sealed the leak
Gastrostomy tube "G" tube	This tube goes into the main body of the stomach. It can be used to keep the stomach decompressed or to feed the patient, or both.	These tubes can be removed anywhere from week 2 and beyond once the patient is doing well.
Jejunostomy tubes	This tube goes into the small bowel and is used to feed the patient	Once the patient is able to take nourishment by mouth these tubes can be removed
G-J tubes	These tubes have a portion in the stomach, to decompress the stomach, and another portion in the small bowel to feed the patient	These are removed when the patient is doing well enough to feed him or herself.

Tube type	Use of the tube	When it is removed
Central line	An intravenous line that goes into a vein in the neck (the jugular) or the chest (the subclavian). They can deliver nutrition much better than a standard IV.	Sometimes these lines are put in at the time of surgery in patients who are "hard sticks." They can be removed at discharge.
PICC lines – Peripherally inserted central catheter. Sometimes placed by a radiologist or a specially trained nurse.	These, like central lines, can be used for nutrition, antibiotics and blood draws.	They can be taken out once the patient no longer needs intravenous access.

Not everyone has all of these tubes and lines, and some of them are only used in patients who have had some problems or difficulties. They are all useful, and they can all be lifesaving. But, you probably really wanted to hear about my Foley catheter.

Foley Catheter

Often a Foley catheter is inserted into your bladder to drain the urine during surgery, sometimes it is inserted later if your plumbing backs up and needs to be drained.

When I had my knee surgery, as you may recall from carefully reading this book, I was on a lot of Demerol and my brother had brought a six-pack of beer. One nurse came by and told me that I shouldn't be drinking while I had the narcotics. I looked up and informed her that I wasn't planning on driving that night. Besides relieving pain, Demerol can keep a sphincter closed. The next morning I woke up and felt as if my bladder was filled with a watermelon. I was in this machine that kept my leg moving, so I called for the nurses to give me a hand. They sent in this tiny little nurse's aid. I told her that I thought if I could just stand up, I could pee in this jug. She dutifully helped me out of the contraption and I leaned on her while holding the jug in the appropriate position.

Thirty minutes passed and this nice lady sighed and said, "Dr. Simpson, I'm getting tired." I knew what had to be done, so told the nurse I would need to have a Foley catheter. Now all of the nurses had known me for years, and perhaps that was the reason, but none of them wanted to put this catheter in me. So, they called the "urology technician." The tech was a nice fellow, had most of his teeth and shaved on alternate weeks. He placed the catheter in me and a liter and a half of urine came out. Everyone knows that a doctor who treats himself has a fool for a patient, and this doctor was no exception. Normally if there is more than 300 cc after placing a catheter it is standard to leave the catheter in for a couple of days—not me. That night the same urology technician had to replace the catheter, and the second time it felt as if someone had made the catheter out of sandpaper.

Stomach Tubes

All the tubes in you will seem to be a bit overwhelming. It is difficult for family members to see tubes of various sorts coming out of their loved ones, but the tubes can be lifesaving.

Tubes in the stomach have one of two uses: either to decompress the stomach, or to feed the patient. If the stomach isn't able to empty it will distend, and early post-operative, a stomach that distends too far inward can rupture at the staple line, causing a leak. Three things cause stomachs to distend: the first is anything that a patient drinks, the second is air that a patient swallows (one reason some surgeons and nurses don't allow you to drink from a straw or swallow ice); and the last reason is that the stomach makes juices (gastric juices). Stomachs don't work well after they have been cut, stapled, or sewed. Most stomachs recover in 24 hours, although some take days or even weeks. This is why some patients have either a G-tube or a nasogastric tube after surgery. While it is inconvenient to have a "nose hose," they do prevent vomiting. It looks cruel but sometimes if a patient has persistent vomiting, placing a nasogastric tube is a kind thing to do.

Some surgeons use no drainage tubes in the stomach whatsoever, and some use more than one tube. If there is a leak, a tube allows the contents to drain out the tube. When the body seals that leak, the tube is removed. While it doesn't always work that way, it does provide a bit of protection. Since leaks occur in one to three percent of patients, some surgeons feel more comfortable having a tube present. Some patients develop an abscess following surgery and a radiologist may need to place a drain into the abscess as a part of the therapy. Occasionally a patient has to be taken back to surgery just to place a drain.

A gastric tube is placed directly into the stomach from the belly wall. For RNY patients, these are placed in the lower pouch. It allows the lower pouch to be decompressed if needed, and the patient can be fed through this tube. If you have a Fobi pouch a G-tube is always placed in the lower pouch.

A jejunostomy tube is placed in the small bowel and the patient is fed through it. If a patient has a leak or is having severe protein malnutrition, this tube provides a safe method for feeding the gut while the body recovers.

The G-J tube is placed in the stomach with an extension into the jejunum. These tubes have two uses: they can decompress the stomach through one port and feed the patient through another port.

IV Tubes

An IV is essential in the hospital, but it is difficult to find a vein in some patients. For these patients, there are two solutions: one is a central line that goes into a large vein in the neck, the chest, or (rarely) in the groin. The other is a PICC line that a specially-trained nurse or a radiologist places. These lines can also be used to feed patients ,where a regular IV in the arm, hand, or leg cannot be used for these special solutions. Often if a patient is a "hard stick" for an IV, I will ask the anesthesiologist to place a central line while we are doing surgery and we remove that line before the patient goes home.

Linguini With Drain Sauce

—how we remove the tubes

Removing any of these tubes is not difficult. Most patients say they feel like linguini is being removed from their body. Usually a bit of local anesthesia is injected at the site of the tube, the suture is cut, the surgeon counts to three and he pulls the drain out. Some tubes have balloons inside of you that are deflated first. Every now and then a tube breaks off, requiring a bit of surgery to get it out, but that is pretty rare. The surgeon usually removes the tube in his office. It is virtually painless but messy, so I give is this advice—if your drain is going to be removed, be sure to wear something old, something you don't care that gets stained.

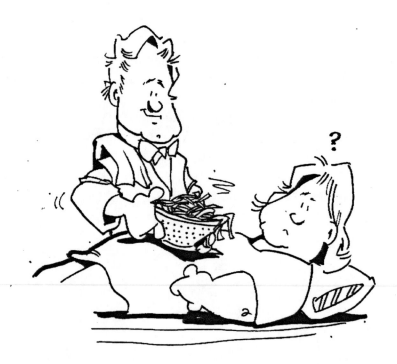

When having a drain removed, be sure to wear old clothes. That way, when they ask what is on your clothes you can say, "drain sauce."

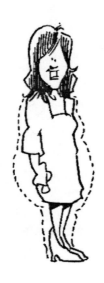

Four

Support Groups

Support Groups, Angels, Internet, and More

There are a lot of reasons to join a support group and to attend the support group meetings, and a lot of reasons that people don't. You can find support after surgery in your surgeon's support group, but also on the internet and through smaller groups of friends. So why attend a support group? Because you are not alone on your weight loss journey, you are not the first person in the world to have bariatric surgery, because you don't need to be ashamed, isolated, or angry at the world because of your obesity. When you make the transition from being morbidly obese to being thin, a lot of things change, and sometimes change is hard to accept and to deal with.

Now, I hate modern psychobabble as much as the next person, but let me say this anyway. Some family and friends are merely enablers of obesity, and as you change your eating habits and your body begins to change, and you go from being shut-in to being more outgoing, your friends and family members may become jealous or upset. Your relationships that were built around lunches of super-sized Big Whoppers and French fries (or Freedom Fries), change as you eat a small bit of tuna fish and avoid the high-carbohydrate, fat-laden foods. They feel they no longer have anything in common with you and they no longer invite you out. (It could also be that watching you eat your tuna and salad makes them feel guilty about all the calories they consume.)

Your support group can become like family. These people know what you are going through. They have already been through it, so they can lend you a shoulder to cry on and some encouragement. They can help you adjust to the changes in your body and your emotions. This might sound a bit new-age for some, but I have not met a patient yet who would not benefit from joining a support group and interacting with other weight loss patients.

Obese people develop many psychological ways of coping with their obesity. Now, I don't want to make broad generalizations (yes, that was a pun) but here are a few observations. There is the "jolly" fat person, the class clown. Al Roker was a master at this. He developed his "jolly" personality, he will tell you, in order to fend off the weight of criticism from his obesity. It was successful for him when he was overweight and even more so after he had weight loss surgery. One of the fears that Al Roker expressed was that, if he lost weight, people would look

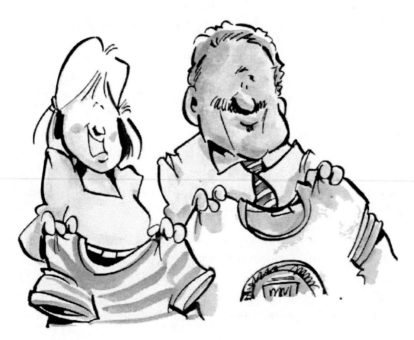

at him differently. He was afraid that the public wouldn't like his newer, thinner self. He worked through this and found his audience loved him just as much after he lost weight.

You will lose some "friends" as you lose weight, but you will gain many more in their place, and these will be people who like the new, slimmer and healthier you. Some interesting changes happen with an obese person's personality when he or she begins to lose weight. Some patients become quite confident and aggressive following surgery, and may exclude family members they once were close to; especially if they realize the family members were enablers.

The divorce rate after this surgery is very high—and there are a lot of theories about this: one lady who had been married for over twenty years said, "I changed, I made the greatest sacrifice I could, undergoing surgery, but he wasn't going to change. He was the same person who still drank too much, and he still abused me. So one day I told him to get out." There are a lot of complex reasons for this. But I have also seen the opposite. One patient who I thought was headed for a divorce before surgery, based on the rather cruel comments she made about her husband, found that after surgery their life changed so much for the better.

Things will change

A lot of things will change: the way you eat, your tastes in food, the way you dress, and your bathroom habits will change. No one will understand you better than someone else who has gone through the surgery. They can give a perspective that I cannot give.

Your support group can help you find new restaurants in your neighborhood that are friendly for weight loss stomachs. They often have great collections of recipes, and more than one person there will offer to pass some clothes on to you as you transition from size 28 to 22 to 10.

Internet Support Groups

The internet provides a great adjunct for a support group. Any day on the message boards for various support groups (OSSG – Obesity Surgery Support Group), there are common and repeated questions. In the chatroom at obesityhelp.com, you will find patients at various places in the weight loss cycle: pre-op, post-op, and long-term post-op. All are anxious to answer questions, give tips, share recipes, and tell you their story.

Remember, besides the questions you will ask at the support group meetings, there are some things you will just need to ask your surgeon or primary care physician. Your doctor should answer questions about your medications, abdominal pain, fevers, or other health matters. Support groups are meant for support, they are not for medical advice. The same goes for the internet chatrooms and support groups. I was in a chatroom when someone asked if it was normal to vomit blood. I said, "No," and asked why. The woman said she had been vomiting blood for a couple of days. I told her to go to the hospital immediately. Luckily, she did, as her blood count was less than half normal and she had a bleeding ulcer. So, when in doubt, seek medical attention.

Roma Downey and *Touched by an Angel:* I loved that show, even though I am not a terribly religious person. In fact, I worry about the lightening that flashes whenever I pass near a church. But angels are something that I believe in. I know a number of them, and anyone who has had, or is going to have this surgery, can become one.

An angel is anyone who visits a patient in the hospital. They can encourage, visit, and be a buddy. They become the nucleus of the support group. Several of my patients started visiting patients even before they had surgery and they continue to do this. One of my patients, Kathy, became so inspired by this that she is starting back to school to become a nurse!

You would be surprised at how much patients appreciate this. Sometimes patients don't want to go to support groups, they don't want to be involved, but when they have surgery, they appreciate a visit from an angel. Anyone who is sick in the hospital loves visitors, but an angel is special. If the angel has gone through surgery he or she can empathize so well with what you are going through, and can tell you what is normal to feel and what is not.

Even more important, they know when to leave. Family members sometimes feel as if they must stay with their mom, spouse, brother or sister twenty-four hours a day. When you are in the hospital, there are times for visitors to be there, and times for them not to be there. Angels know this, especially if they have been through the surgery. Sometimes the visits are only 15 minutes, but it means so much to the patient to have that time. So, if you have your surgery and someone says they will be your angel, please let them. They can help and encourage more than you know. Many life-long friendships have been developed from this.

In our age of the internet, there are even internet angels! They will collect well wishes from all those who know them on the chatroom and forward them on to you. While it is not the same as having someone visit you in the hospital, it does connect you with a worldwide support group.

Anyone who is sick in the hospital loves visitors, but an angel is special.

Weight loss surgery is more than just an operation. You have the opportunity to give back and to help others. You will get more out of being an angel than you can ever imagine. That nice little light shining on an angel's head?—well, I cannot promise that you will have one, but you can still be an angel.

When you think of goals for your new life after surgery, please think about helping those who are going through this. You might be shy, and not want to go to support group, you might only be able to give a kind word, or post a simple message, or tell your story. There are many ways, but tell your story. Someone wants to hear it. Someone is going to be where you were—so, give back.

Part 3

Early Post-Op

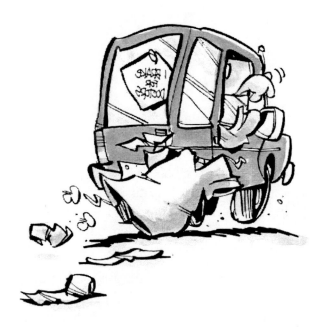

One

The First Twelve Weeks

You are home—you made it. You are in the first twelve weeks of a post-operative period, and the first twelve weeks suck.

Really, they are not fun. Sure, you have read about people who have undergone weight loss surgery and report that it is a walk in the park—they are not normal, they are the exception, and they seem to write a lot on internet bulletin boards.

The first thing you notice is that you hurt a bit more at home than you did in the hospital. In the hospital you had a nurse and host of other people to take care of your needs. Perhaps you didn't like the way they took care of you, but you didn't have to worry about anything but getting up and doing laps around the nurses' station. At home it is a different matter, especially if you have kids (and that includes a husband who, after all, is just a larger version of a child).

Sleep

—No, You Don't Need a Pill

Sleep disturbances after any major surgery are common. In fact sleeping in general is a difficult problem. Remember the nurses waking you up to take blood pressure, check on your pulse, and in general ask you a few questions? Remember your roommate, or the fellow across the hall that loved to yell out for Aunt Mabel? When sleep cycles become disturbed, it is difficult to get them back. Do not fret, your only goal during this period of time is to keep fluids in and walk. Sleeping pills are not the answer, and may be a problem, and pain medication taken in order to sleep is definitely not the answer.

Sleeping pills are highly addictive and the quality of sleep is not that good.

Sleeping pills are highly addictive, and the quality of sleep is not that good. Some studies have shown that you become dependent on the pills for sleep in a very short period of time, so my policy has been to never prescribe them.

Some patients use the narcotic to help them sleep but that has the same effect: the sleep you get will be poor, and the ability to sleep without the pills becomes more difficult.

If you are going to be up in the night what should you do? If you want to be sleeping then you shouldn't reward yourself by watching television, hanging out in internet chatrooms, or reading a good book. Instead, follow the Christian Harris plan: if you have not fallen asleep in 45 minutes then get up and do something you do not like to do. For example, if you hate washing the dishes, then wash them or clean up something, scrub the kitchen floor, whatever. Do that for 45 minutes and go back to bed. If you still cannot go to sleep, then repeat what you did—yes, that means, re-wash the dishes. Again—for 45 minutes. You don't get the feeling you have accomplished anything, and it isn't fun. Eventually your body will get the joke and simply sleep. If in several weeks you have another bout with insomnia, get up and wash the dishes.

I gave the Harris prescription to a very nice young housewife who immediately started to laugh at me. She said, "You really don't know me, do you, Dr.

Simpson?" I told her that I didn't understand, and she said the thing she enjoyed the most was cleaning, putting things in order, categorizing, and would happily spend the entire evening rewashing dishes. I didn't want to give her the diagnosis of obsessive-compulsive-disorder (OCD) since she had already given it to herself. My next immediate thought was to hire her to do the filing in my office; she could have the night shift. She did find a task she didn't like doing, and before long was enjoying a restful night's sleep. The task that got her to sleep was reading her daughter's homework in history.

The other way to break a simple cycle of staying up too late isn't something you can do right after surgery—to pull and all-nighter and go to bed the following evening at a reasonable hour.

Getting Into and Out of Bed

–and other places to sleep

Getting in and out of bed can be a major challenge. It isn't fun, it isn't easy, and the more pain you feel in your incision, the harder it is. For most patients we recommend you obtain a recliner to sleep in the first few nights. It is easier to get in and out of them, and they can be quite comfortable. Some recliners take a lot of work to get in and out of, so if you are in the market for one, make certain the one you purchase glides easily. There are even recliners that have the electronic helper to get you out of them. I always imagine these devices going crazy and launching a patient into orbit.

Be sure and have some favorite items on the nightstand: a sports bottle with water, a telephone (lighted) and easy access to the bathroom. Some patients like keeping their pain medicine by their nightstand, and if you feel you need to that is fine, but if you do, I recommend keeping only one dose by your nightstand. Why?—Because that way you don't have to worry about overdosing yourself in your sleep. If your spouse puts a lot of pain medicine by your nightstand—be very worried.

Oh, if you need to get up and go to the bathroom, get up and go. Don't have a urinal there; especially don't keep it by the sports bottle! You need to walk, so think about getting up and walking.

Other patients purchase pillow wedges so they have some elevation by their bed. Still others make these wedges with lots of pillows surrounding them (reminds me of a cocoon). Having a hospital bed can help the first couple of days, but very few patients get these, and they are rarely needed. I often wish I had one so I could sit up and watch my favorite television program at night. We do like patients to sleep at a fifteen-degree upright angle, and for some the only way is to have the head of your bed propped up a bit. This is one of those little chores you should do before you go to the hospital.

Feeling Tired and Needing Naps

Surgery is tough. You will need naps and you will be very tired if you return to work after three weeks. There is nothing wrong with you, you had major surgery, and major surgery takes a lot out of you. Expect that it will be three months before you feel normal.

Taking naps is normal after major surgery; so if you feel like it, don't deny yourself. You need to follow a few simple rules about naptime, however. First, if you are going to take a nap, then take a nap. Don't sit in your recliner watching re-runs and drifting in and out of sleep. Do like President Harry Truman did, undress, go to bed, turn out the light, and take a proper nap. Don't take a long nap either; twenty minutes to an hour is all that you will need, not a two or four-hour rest. If you take longer naps, you will have difficulty resting throughout the night.

Those who have had laparoscopy surgery have the same metabolic effects of open surgery: the changes in your own body's metabolism are all unrelated to whether the surgery was done "open" or laparoscopically. So, plan on three months during which you will feel a bit tired. While it will get better, it gets better on a week-to-week basis, not day-to-day, so you will notice that this week you feel a bit better than last week. Mondays however, especially when you go back to work, still feel like Mondays, no matter how much weight you lose, and Fridays, well, they are still a great day.

Why Can't I Concentrate?

—or, just hand me the comics

Your ability to concentrate on even simple things following surgery is impaired. This is one of the reasons we ask you to have affairs in order prior to surgery, because after surgery it is sometimes difficult to concentrate. This became clear to me after having some knee surgery a number of years ago. I remember going home and instead of reading the newspaper, one of my favorite activities, all I could do was look at the pictures. I knew my ability to concentrate was not very good when some politicians actually made sense to me.

This is a temporary condition. You are not becoming senile; it is simply another effect of surgery. The best way to overcome this is to do plenty of walking, keep drinking water, and if you find that my book becomes funnier after surgery, then you are the exception and your ability to reason has improved.

Eating and Puking

There are those patients who wake up, have stomachs made of steel, and seem to have no problem eating anything from the third day on after surgery. Then there are those patients for whom eating is a very unpleasant and difficult experience, and will continue to be so for the first twelve weeks.

There is a whole section in this book about nausea and vomiting, but essentially it boils down to this: if you vomit, stop eating and drinking for a while—give your stomach a rest. Then resume a clear liquid diet.

Don't give up on any foods. There are foods that suit your stomach better immediately after surgery, but one day tuna fish may not do well, and the next day tuna fish may do just great.

Nausea

Nausea is common the first few weeks after surgery. Your stomach was sutured, it is painful, it wants to rebel, and it will. Most nausea comes from overfilling your stomach with too much food or fluid. Once the stomach distends, it feels uncomfortable and you feel nauseated. When the stomach becomes more filled it will produce more acid. The more acid in your stomach, the less your stomach likes it. Overfilling the stomach, and too much acid, both cause severe nausea. When you are nauseated you may also find certain odors bother you (cigarettes, cheap perfume, your mother-in-law's cooking).

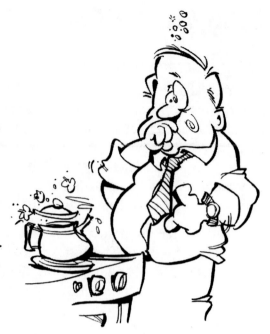

- Remember the size of your stomach and do not over fill it. (Simpson Commandment Number One.)

- Take the Pepcid® or Zantac® daily (or Nexium®, Prevacid®, etc.) Pepcid Complete® is a great product that allows you to have immediate relief from stomach acid as well as keeping acid decreased later.

- Keep something in your stomach. Some of our patients have found that Matzos works well (it can be found in the international food section of most supermarkets). Matzos have little salt, and are rather bland. But every pregnant woman will tell you that a soda cracker soaks up acid and can help with nausea. Remember, this is early in the post-operative period, the first twelve weeks. We do not expect that crackers, which are a high-carbohydrate food, will be a part of your daily food.

- Odors can cause nausea. Your husband or wife will have to smoke outside. My patients refer to this as the bionic nose.

- Some herbal teas help with nausea, such as Lemon Lift, Peppermint, or Ginger. But if you overfill your stomach or pouch with tea you will defeat its purpose.

- Friends will tell you to drink some Seven-Up or ginger ale. Avoid these and all carbonated beverages. Avoid these well-meaning people also: they are evil and trying to destroy you (just kidding). Some surgeons believe that carbonation can stretch the stomach and even disrupt staples during the early post-operative period. There is little evidence to prove this, but unless your surgeon says it is okay, don't do it. While carbonation may work fine in some stomachs, you have to remember, your stomach now contains a lot less space.

- The narcotics in pain medicine can cause nausea. Codeine and Percocet® are two of the more common ones. Sometimes patients have to simply avoid narcotics and use Tylenol® for pain.

- Keep drinking fluids. Your goal is 2 quarts a day (about 2 liters is fine). Sip. But remember, you do not have to drink all of this at once. Keeping a sports bottle filled with water is a good thing to do.

Vomiting

Vomiting is awful. Often it happens because you overeat. You have a limited amount of room, and if your stomach does not empty fast enough, you will distend the stomach and you will vomit. So you must learn portion control. If your stomach holds four ounces, that is eight tablespoons. If you have one teaspoon too much you can feel awful and vomit. You may stay nauseated all day long, and you may not be able to hold food down.

Remember do not eat and drink at the same time early on. When you had a 50-oz stomach this was okay, but fluids fill your DS 4-oz stomach very fast and a RNY or Lap band one-ounce stomach even faster (one medicine cup or shot glass is one ounce). If you eat a couple of ounces of food and then drink some water you can quickly over-fill your stomach. These rules can change after a while; we are talking the first few weeks here.

Vomiting can become a cycle. If you keep vomiting, the outlet from your stomach can swell, obstructing your stomach and causing more vomiting. This can either be the stoma (in the case of the RNY or lap-band), the pylorus, or any portion of the stomach. Sometimes we have to put patients in the hospital and give them intravenous fluids because of intractable vomiting. Often, if we limit the amount they can take by mouth and go back to clear liquids we can stop the vomiting. If you are having trouble with nausea and vomiting do this:

- Stop drinking and eating for a while. If you keep drinking or eating, and then vomiting you will only cause swelling that will prevent the normal passage of fluid. After you feel better, you can gently begin clear liquids. Just like when you have the flu, it is okay to skip fluids for several hours.

- Go back to clear liquids only. Start by drinking a teaspoon-full every five minutes while you are awake. This should keep you hydrated and not over-do it. If you keep hydrated, you will not need to go into the hospital. If you feel full or become nauseated with drinking, **STOP**.

- Protein intake is a key to success with these operations. Isopure® and other protein drinks are clear liquids and count toward the two liters a day. But remember, protein is a goal to get to. You do not have to "stuff" protein in the first few weeks. The goal is to get your stomach working, then once it is, to put protein first.

- Suck on ice cubes, or make some Popsicle (Isopure® in the ice cube tray (diluted with some water) will help you a lot). Do not use sugar-filled popsicles.

- Keep track of how much you drink at a time. Measure it. If you feel full, don't drink. After surgery, surgeons will have measured your stomach size and will tell you how large it is. Do not exceed that amount. Often nausea and vomiting will happen if you drink too much too fast. We want you to sip water like it is fine Kentucky bourbon.

- Remember, if your stomach will not empty fast and you keep putting fluid in it, you will vomit. So drink SLOWLY. If you feel full, DO NOT DRINK—it is not worth it to vomit.

You may be given a prescription for Reglan® to help empty your stomach. Some patients find that liquid Reglan works better than pills. Reglan works particularly well for patients who have diabetes, as they might have a "diabetic gastropathy," which essentially means your stomach doesn't empty well. This condition usually improves with time.

Once you are feeling better you may advance your diet gently. Remember, when you vomit, we go back to the beginning, just like in the hospital. Stop eating, wait a while, begin a few clear liquids and go from there.

Sometimes patients vomit because they try something that does not agree with them. Usually this is meat. The stomach, at first, may have a difficult time digesting certain meats and vegetables. This is why we advocate that you add one thing new to your diet per day. If something does not agree with you today, try it later. Red meat takes some patients three months before they can tolerate it—except for Tammy. Tammy on her fourth post-operative day was given beef tips. Sure enough, she ate them. She did very well in her post-operative period, and was able to get to her goal in a year.

If all this fails, call your surgeon. If you can only keep water down we need to know. This is usually an exaggeration, and your surgeon will want to hear what you can keep down, and what you cannot. If you can only keep water down, then it is fine to drink only water for a couple of days. You will not melt away. If you truly cannot keep anything down your surgeon will want you in the hospital.

Remember; just because you have this surgery does not make you immune from the flu, stomach viruses, food poisoning, bowel obstruction, or a host of other problems. Do not hesitate to talk to your family physician regarding your vomiting, especially if the flu is going around. If you are having vomiting and diarrhea, you may need intravenous fluids sooner rather than later.

Warning—Preventable Brain Damage

Repeated vomiting episodes can quickly lead to a vitamin deficiency that can cause brain damage, a peripheral neuropathy, and muscle wasting. This can be prevented with vitamin repletion. While hospitalized, it is important to have IV fluids with the yellow stuff (multivitamins) in it, especially if you have been admitted more than two times for dehydration. If you are in another city or are being admitted by different doctors for dehydration, be sure to ask that they include multivitamins with their intravenous hydration.

Other Stomach Problems

Heartburn

Heartburn occurs when the acid from your stomach goes up into your esophagus and burns it. This is also known as Gastro-esophageal reflux disease (GERD). If you overfill your stomach, you will have GERD. There is a bit more to reflux disease than this. Obesity is related to reflux, so is pregnancy (the excess weight presses on the diaphragm). The first twelve weeks after surgery is when most patients experience this. RNY patients have an advantage in that reflux is essentially cured by this operation. There are some simple things you can do to prevent GERD (heartburn):

- Fluid and food portion control (see Simpson commandment number one)

- Elevate the head of your bed about 15 degrees. Many of you will sleep in a recliner the first couple of weeks. Some of you will use pillow wedges in bed, and others will have elevated hospital beds.

- Caffeine, alcohol, and chocolate increase GERD by relaxing the sphincter between the stomach and the esophagus. During the first twelve weeks you may not want to be consuming the alcohol or chocolate anyway. Norwegians are allowed coffee.

- Carbonated beverages are forbidden by some surgeons. No plop plop, fizz, fizz for you. But these beverages can exacerbate reflux.

- You may need to add Reglan® at night along with the Pepcid. You may need some stronger medicine, such as Prevacid, Nexium, etc.

- Tums, or better yet, Pepcid Complete, gives you immediate relief from the acid and also a longer-term relief.

Diarrhea

–or, keeping it loose

Not only can high protein keep your stools loose, so can your new anatomy. Four loose stools a day is common for duodenal switch or a long-limb Roux-en-Y bypass. You may need to bulk up your diet with soluble fiber such as Citrucel®, or a generic-based methylcellulose. We don't recommend psillium seed products as they can cause gas. Milk products can also cause diarrhea after surgery, anytime guts are rearranged patients can find themselves intolerant of lactose. If you have black stools, if you have blood in your stools, or if the diarrhea persists for more than two days, call your surgeon. DO NOT, on your own, take products to stop the diarrhea.

If you have an antibiotic-associated colitis, taking Kaopectate or Lomotle can make it much worse. But diarrhea is a matter of degree. Some patients think having loose stools is considered diarrhea, but surgeons don't think that way. Two large-volume very loose stools is considered diarrhea. Some surgeons, myself included, have patients undergo a bowel prep before surgery (vodka and Golytely is called the Simpson cocktail). Sometimes this prep solution is still in the patient for a while after surgery, so their first bowel movement can be explosive. Fats, which are not digested well in distal bypass patients, can cause diarrhea.

Constipation

–sung to Carly Simon's "anticipation"

Constipation is not fun—it is awful, and it is a common problem with proximal RNY, VBG, and lap-band. The answer is always the same, it never varies: you need to drink more water. Of course, everyone tells me that they drink "gallons" of water and that it doesn't help. Simply put: your colon absorbs water, and it will absorb more water as you need of it. If you drink a lot of water, then it won't absorb as much and you will have looser stools. The second solution is soluble fiber. We recommend fiber that is based on methylcellulose (like Citrucel® that you can purchase in a sugar-free variety). In fact, we also recommend fiber for patients who have loose stools as it will helps "bulk" them up a bit. So, fiber and water are the keys. Oh, one more thing—walk! The more you walk, the better the bowels move. The less you walk, the slower your bowels get. So, water, walk, and fiber. Do not start taking laxatives—you can become dependent upon them and they are not something you wish to become dependent upon. Have a glass of Citrucel and take a brisk walk.

Hemorrhoids – a Real Pain In the...

A hemorrhoid is a painful complex of veins in the rectum that can cause bleeding, itching, soiling and even pain. Some say they are varicose veins of the rectum caused by abnormal straining. This is caused by two conditions—diarrhea and constipation. If you bring reading material into the bathroom with you, then you are setting yourself up for hemorrhoids. Preventing them is simple: have fiber and water. The answer is the same for both diarrhea and constipation. For both, you need to have more soluble fiber to bulk up the stools and you need to increase your water intake. We recommend a methylcellulose fiber such as Citrucel, as it causes less gas than fiber made from seeds.

There are a few things that you can do to help relieve the symptoms from hemorrhoids. First, though, we recommend that you see your surgeon to make certain that your problem is a hemorrhoid and not something else that needs treatment. Tucks® are a great product. Use them according to the directions, and you will find a lot of relief from the pain, swelling and itching from hemorrhoids. There are various creams and ointments for the treatment of hemorrhoids but often the over-the-counter medications just don't work that well. A sitz bath is a device you can find at many pharmacies that allows you to soak your backside in some nice warm water. Some like it hot, some like it cold, and some like it warm. It doesn't matter what the temperature of the water is that you use in the sitz bath. Use what feels good and take them often, but limit them to 20 minutes at a time. Sometimes you need to have surgery for the hemorrhoids, and if that thought doesn't get you to use fiber and water, remember that after the surgery you will be using the stuff anyway.

Flatulence

Everyone does it. In the hospital I ask daily if patients have passed flatus, and they are quite happy to report it when they do. However, outside the hospital people are not so happy to be passing gas. Gas comes from two sources: swallowed air, and bacteria in your gut that is breaking down some food that your body doesn't digest. The foods that are known to cause most gasses are beans (shocking), some fruits, soft drinks, whole grains/wheat and bran, milk and milk products, foods containing sorbitol and dietetic products.

Devrom® or Nullo® can help eliminate some odors. You can order Devrom at (800) 453-8898, or their website htp://www.parthenoninc.com.

Hernia

If you feel a bulge under your incision, you might have a hernia. If the bulge comes out when you strain, lift, or cough, and goes back in when you lay down, you probably have a hernia and your surgeon will want to see you in the office to confirm it. Hernias become larger with time and will need repair. They do not improve on their own, no exercise will help them, they will grow, they will get worse, and they can cause a problem. Sometimes the hernia, or bulge, does not go back—and we have a cute term for that—incarcerated (as in jail).

Hernias can be painful but usually they are not. Sometimes you strain your incision when you lift things, and if you do, you need to give your muscles a rest: a strain is not a hernia. The pain from a hernia can be sharp or it can be a dull ache that feels worse at the end of the day. Remember, your fascia (gristle) is what holds you together and after surgery your stomach is held together by sutures that are as strong as a thirty-pound test fishing line. Those sutures are strongest when they are first put in and dissolve over time, and at the same time your body is healing that fascia together. Some surgeons use permanent sutures that do not dissolve over time, but these do not guarantee that a hernia will not develop.

Often hernias happen about a month after surgery when people feel fine and then lift something heavy. The most common patients who develop hernias are mothers; it is hard to resist picking up your child, especially a month after surgery when you are feeling better. If you have a hernia it will only become larger with time, and you will need to have surgery. If you have a hernia, and you suddenly develop pain, nausea and vomiting, call your surgeon immediately; do not wait for an appointment.

My mentor in surgery was a great surgeon named George Block. He closed all abdominal incisions with wire on the inside. When you learned to tie the wire suture, you passed his rotation, I really loved Dr. Block and became a surgeon because of him, but I hated tying wire sutures.

Other Problems

Yeast Infections/Thrush

Some patients are prone to a yeast infection, which either manifests itself as thrush (a painful white coating of the tongue) or as a rash under the armpits, in the groin area or in the skin. These happen for a variety of reasons; the most common reason is antibiotic use. The antibiotics wipe out "friendly" bacteria that inhabit the skin and mouth and other places, allowing yeast to take over. When I had knee surgery they used a single dose of antibiotics and I developed the worst case of jock itch—another fungus. There are some over-the-counter products for this and prescriptions are available for severe cases.

Hair Today, Gone Tomorrow

Hair thinning or loss is expected after rapid weight loss. There are those who firmly believe that taking protein, biotin or other vitamins and supplements, prevents this. Some hair loss is associated with zinc deficiency, protein deficiency and other deficiencies of vitamins and minerals, but this is a rare contributing factor to post-operative patients' hair loss. For those thirty percent who have hair loss, the hair will come back fuller and richer than before. No shampoo will prevent it, but perms and coloring may accelerate hair loss during this time.

The realm of hair-care products, the amount of things that salons put into your hair and scalp, remind me of toxic waste dumps. It makes me wonder why more people don't lose their hair. I mean think about it: people with curly hair have products designed to straighten their hair, people with straight hair get stuff to curl their hair, if you are blonde you want to be more blonde or a red-head, if you are auburn or brown you want to be blonde or black, and if you are grey—well, then all is lost and it is time to find out what Clairol has to make your hair any color but that.

Hair loss is caused from the hair follicles resetting themselves in the face of the stress of surgery, weight loss, and other factors we do not understand. There are a lot of products on the store shelves that claim to prevent hair loss. You can spend your money on these products but I would prefer you purchase this book, become educated and support my pocket instead of your local hairdresser's.

Sexuality

You may resume sexual activity when you feel up to it, usually seventeen years after surgery (sorry, couldn't resist). Don't forget birth control. We would like you to wait two years before getting pregnant. For birth control during this time we recommend a diaphragm, condoms, an IUD, or even the patch, but not the pill. Some oral contraceptives are not absorbed well after this surgery. Planning for your pregnancy is better than being surprised and naming the child after your favorite surgeon.

Pregnancy

As stated above, we recommend that you avoid this issue so use birth control religiously (Okay, there are some who would have a problem with that, so for those, just avoid). You may start planning a pregnancy after 12 months, although most surgeons prefer for you to wait 24 months to conceive. If you become pregnant, we will need to enlist the aid of a good OB doctor.

The period of rapid weight loss during your first post-operative year is not a healthy time to nourish a fetus. Children are a great addition to most families, and I am very pro-kids (no, I am not available for baby sitting and I do not want to borrow your teenager). There are many patients who undergo weight loss surgery specifically to have children, and to those of you who fit into this category—good luck.

Returning to Work

Some patients return to work on a part-time basis in as little as two weeks after surgery, most return to work after three weeks. If you do a lot of lifting and cannot get a light duty status, you may need to be out of work for as long as six weeks after surgery. Your workplace probably has forms for your surgeon to fill out for you to return to work. There is a lot on those forms for you to fill out and it is always helpful to do that—for example, your name, your address, the date you had your surgery. One time a patient faxed us five pages of these government-issued blank forms. The patient didn't fill out his name or any information, nor did his fax have a return number on it. The patient became irate that we had not filled them out until he realized that we had no idea who had faxed them to us. Please fill out as much as possible before your surgeon's office staff sees them. Also, ask for an extra copy—things do get lost.

Driving

No, you cannot drive home from the hospital

There are a few simple rules about when you can drive. First, if you are taking narcotics, pain pills such as Vicodin, Percocet, Davocet, you should not drive a car. If you drive under the influence of these drugs you can be arrested, put in jail, have your license suspended, and may injure yourself or someone else. Second, you shouldn't drive until your reaction time has returned to normal. Have you ever been driving along and suddenly notice the person in front of you has stopped? You have to slam on your brakes and just avoid rear-ending them. Well, imagine if your reaction time is one second off—instead of just barely missing the car in front of you, you now have your engine in your lap.

If the thought of slamming on your brakes makes your incision hurt, then you shouldn't be driving. Some surgeons want patients to wait two or three weeks, but there are clearly some patients who should wait even longer. I had knee surgery in 1989, and my friends tell me it is still too early for me to drive.

What About Bathing, Swimming, Jacuzzi???

The decision on when to resume these activities is best left up to the surgeon. Most surgeons want patients to wait for three weeks before baptism.

When to Call Your Surgeon

Call your surgeon when:

- pus comes out of the wound

- the wound becomes progressively more red

- red streaks run from the wound

- the wound becomes unusually tender

- your temperature is greater than 101 degrees F

- you have yellow or green FOUL-smelling drainage

Some clear yellow drainage from your wound is normal. This liquid is generally liquefied fat cells that were destroyed when we made our grand entrance into your body.

Things you can and cannot do to the wound

- It is okay to allow soap and water to run over the wound

- Do not use Neosporin® or other ointments on the wound

- Do not bathe or swim for three weeks

- If you are outside in the sun, the wound will burn easily, so keep it covered

- After several weeks it is okay to use sunblock on the wound

Wound Infections

If you have a wound infection your doctor, or a nurse, will give you instructions about how to take care of the wound. Generally, the wound is packed with saltwater-soaked gauze and this dressing is changed a couple of times a day. Antibiotics are prescribed, typically Keflex® or Augmentin® (unless you have an allergy to these). An infection usually comes from bacteria that live on your skin. It rarely that comes from a dirty instrument in the operating room or some other source. This is why it is important to keep your wound clean.

If your wound has been opened to allow the pus to drain, it is still advisable to wash your wound with soap and water—it won't hurt the wound and it is the best thing for it. Once the wound infection has healed and the wound looks healthy, the surgeon may close the wound with sutures or he may wait until the wound closes by itself. Sometimes these wound infections can take weeks to heal completely, so be patient. This does not mean that you will need to be on antibiotics for all this time. If the surrounding skin doesn't show red streaking, chances are the surgeon will take you off the antibiotics.

Packing a wound

Your surgeon will have you "pack" the wound with some saline-soaked gauze. Please do not stuff this in the wound—the idea is for the wound edges to remain moist. If you stuff gauze into the wound, it will take longer for the wound to close. Over time, this wound will start "contracting" and closing itself, and after a few months, no one will notice a difference. But, if you stuff the wound with the gauze instead of layering it over the wound, it will take the wound a lot longer to close. So, be gentle.

Some surgeons use other materials to soak the wound. Some use a weak bleach or iodine solution, acetic acid, or one of a number of other solutions. The important principles are to pack the wound lightly, change the dressing twice a day (unless otherwise instructed) and take a shower. Likewise, there are a number of other products that surgeons can use, such as the wound vac, various forms of gels, or even material from algae (Sorbsan®). These all come with special instructions and will probably also come with a home health nurse to help you manage all of this material. Fear not, if you eat well and consume adequate protein, your wound will close nicely and look just fine.

Wound infections are common and happen about five percent of the time. These infections can be small and easy to manage, or your entire wound might be opened up and allowed to close on its own. If your wound is left to close on its own, a binder sometimes helps. The forces on most wounds are from side to side, tending to keep the wound open longer. Check with your surgeon—he or she may have other ideas.

Closing a Wound

Sometimes a surgeon will take you back to the operating room to close the wound. This only happens after the wound is very well-healed and has a nice red bit of "granulation" tissue in it. Sometimes a surgeon will allow the wound to slowly close by itself. That your surgeon's decision.

What Suture Did They Use?

There are a lot of ways for a surgeon to close the skin, and a lot of tools. There are advantages and disadvantages to all of them. Skin staples are the least painful, and lead to a good cosmetic result, although a number of patients don't like them. Most surgeons use a dissolving suture and then place steri-strip tapes over the wound. These steri-strips are a wound closure device and some of them are as strong as suture. Still other surgeons use Demabond®, which is superglue for the skin. There is no right or wrong way to close a wound, but there are a lot of opinions. One friend of mine said that in her part of the country, surgeons don't use staples because patients think they are not cosmetically appropriate. No matter where you live or how your wound is closed, it probably will not affect how the wound looks later on.

Why Do I Have this Big Ugly Scar?

Different people scar differently. Some people develop thick ugly scars, which are called keloids, and sometimes those scars have to be revised or removed. Typically, this happens to people who have a lot of pigment in their skin.

The scar will look its worst about six months to a year after surgery. There are several reasons for this. Your body is constantly remodeling itself—worse than a Beverly Hills househusband. As time goes on, your scar will shrink and it will begin to look better. After a couple of years the scar will pretty much look the way it will always look.

Scars respond to motion and forces. For example, scars on joints tend to be thicker because the joint is always moving (very seldom will you find a pretty scar on a knee). In patients with large abdomens, the scars can be very thick because the force of the abdomen is from side to side, and if you have a scar in the middle (up and down) it will tend to become thick. Here is where plastic surgeons always look good. After we bariatric surgeons do the great job of rearranging guts, and the patient loses the weight, the plastic surgeons do their tuck and nip and patients have smaller scars. Perhaps I went in the wrong field. Another reason some weight loss surgeons like their patients to wear a binder for several weeks after the surgery is that it decreases the forces on the incision.

Someone always wants to sell you something to make your scar look better. It might be vitamin E-based, aloe vera-based, or some entirely new brew from their cauldron. There is no evidence that any of this stuff works terribly well. But the rules for your scar are simple: don't put anything on it the first few weeks. always keep it out of the sun (certainly for the first couple of years), and don't ever be afraid of soap and water. Wound infection or not, soap and water will not hurt you—honestly.

Non-prescription Medicines

Over-the-counter: what can I take when I get a cold, or the flu?

There are a few simple rules with weight loss surgery, and one of them is to learn about your body and the medicines you put into it. If you have a cold or the flu and want to take something, remember: if you take something for it, it will take about a week to get over it, but if you take nothing, it will take seven days. Tylenol is okay to take, but it is also found in many other cold and flu medications so be careful to read the label of every medicine you take and do not exceed the maximum daily dose of Tylenol (acetaminophen). Many cold and flu remedies are time-released, and if you have had a bypass surgery, you may not absorb a portion of that time-released medicine so it will be wasted (Contact tablets, for example, will not work well with patients who had a duodenal switch). Some surgeons do not want their patients to take non-steroidal anti-inflammatory medications, such as Motrin or Aspirin, and you should have a list of these, if that is the rule.

Prescription Medications

Again, know what you are taking and why, and avoid time-released medications if you have had a distal bypass. If you have had a proximal bypass you should be monitored carefully by your primary care doctor to make certain that you are getting a therapeutic effect from your medications.

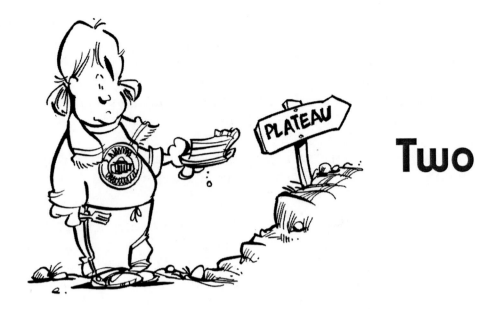

Plateaus

What Is a Plateau?

Every patient stops losing weight after weight loss surgery and wonders why. Often they think their stomach has stretched. Often they just don't know why they stop losing. But first let us define a true plateau. A plateau is when you have maintained your weight and your measurements for four weeks. If you are still losing inches, you are not on a plateau. You are simply redistributing the weight.

The First Six Weeks After Surgery

You will reach a plateau during the first few weeks after surgery. Some people find they weigh more when they come back from the hospital than when they went in. This is usually because a lot of the fluid we pumped in you is still in your tissues, so the first few pounds you lose are typically water weight. The first six weeks after surgery is a fun time, and it is common for patients to lose ten percent of their weight during this time. This means that if you weigh 300 pounds you will lose 30 pounds or more. More is good. Some patients don't have a scale or they are looking forward to the time when their scale can weigh them. You will sometimes lose inches before you lose pounds, as your body is changing where it puts the fat and muscle. It is important to know where you are losing weight. That is why you should take your measurements—as well as your photograph—prior to going to the hospital. So, measure your neck, chest, waist, thighs, and arms before going to surgery, and keep watching those at least once a month.

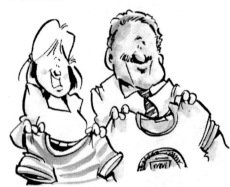

One of my patients didn't have a lot of spending money and didn't want to buy too many clothes until she had a more stable weight. She changed her mind after her underwear fell off at the checkout counter as she was purchasing food in the grocery store. Taking measurements not only helps you chart your progress, it can prevent an embarrassing moment.

Sometime during this first six weeks, the weight loss will stop for a while. Your body is readjusting—that is all. If your surgeon has placed you on a liquid diet, you will also notice that you can drink a lot more than you thought you could. No, you didn't stretch it. It is just that liquids are able to flow passively through the stoma or the pylorus (if you had a duodenal switch). Sometimes you are left with a lot of hunger. In the beginning, fluids will fill your pouch or stomach and you will have little appetite, but as you move forward, you will rediscover your appetite—not a bad thing. This is just one sign that it is time to move to more solid foods.

A readjustment period for the body is necessary. During the post-operative time, you not only lose weight from fat cells, but also from what we call "lean body mass." That is, you lose weight also from muscles. You need this muscle mass for walking, moving around, breathing, and assorted other body functions. That muscle mass needs to be rebuilt, therefore we want you to start a walking program. The more you walk, the more lean body mass you will keep. If you don't use muscle, you will lose it—so start walking.

The Carbohydrate Trap

Surgeons have their own version of a post-operative diet. Some surgeons do not want you eating any sugar-filled foods after surgery, and some surgeons do not mind for the first few weeks. Essentially, the first goal is to get your stomach working again and your body used to its new anatomy. Some items "go down" well, and a lot of things do not. If your surgeon is liberal the first few weeks after surgery, do not assume this is license to continue consuming these types of carbohydrates later on.

This is the carbohydrate trap: you begin to consume juices, yogurt, mashed potatoes—all items that have nutritional value, but also contain a fair bit of calories in the form of carbohydrates. As you transition out of your first few weeks and into "normal" eating, some of those foods should be put aside in favor of low fat, high-quality protein foods. There is nothing wrong with yogurt, fruit juices, or even mashed potatoes. The trouble is that it is possible to consume them in large quantities, even with a small stomach. If your surgeon is lenient in the first few weeks after surgery, remember, these are just transitional "soft" foods; you should not consume them after the "soft" food phase of your diet.

The best example of this is the clear liquid diet. Even patients with diabetes are allowed a clear liquid diet. Many of the approved liquids contain sugar. Immediately after surgery, patients with diabetes are allowed any clear liquid—as the affect of the sugar on their blood sugar level will be minimal. However, when their stomach has fully regained function and they can consume larger quantities of liquids, the types of clear liquids are restricted. That is because if you consume enough of those sugar-filled liquids, your blood sugar can rise. Again—small quantities of almost any food or liquid is fine. However, some patients find that they can consume vast quantities of these "soft" foods and it becomes a trap.

So, beware: as you transition from early post-op period (the first 6-12 weeks) to the later period, you need to limit the "soft" high-carbohydrate foods and move to a higher-protein food.

High-glycemic Index Carbohydrates

Every morning when you consider breakfast you have a choice. You can have the Pop-tart® or you can have an egg with a bit of fruit. Both have 25 grams of carbohydrates (not from the egg but from the fruit), but there is a difference. If you eat the Pop-tart, your blood sugar will quickly rise, which will cause you to produce more insulin, and in a couple of hours, you will be hungry again. If you eat the egg and a bit of fruit (an apple), your blood sugar won't rise as fast, and your sense of "satiety" or fullness will last longer. Glycemic Index is a measure of how fast blood sugar rises after eating carbohydrates. A Pop-tart has a glycemic index of around 70, while an apple has about 28. The higher the glycemic index, the more that food is associated with obesity, diabetes, heart disease, and even cancer. Besides, the apple will have more fiber, more vitamins, and more other good stuff. Although the Pop-tart sounds good, you have the choice of eating what you want or gaining weight. The egg contains protein and has a glycemic index of almost zero.

Carbohydrates are complex molecules of sugar. Some are put together in such a way that the body processes them differently and therefore, they are not associated with as much obesity. Naturally, anything you eat in excess can cause obesity (yes, even if you are on the Atkins diet you can still eat enough fat that your high school outfit will never fit). Carbohydrates that are less likely to cause obesity are vegetables, pulpy fruits (like grapefruit) and legumes. Those most often associated with obesity are breads, rice, pasta, and candy.

While counting carbohydrates is an easy way to lose weight. Remember, those that have a lower-glycemic index are far better for you and will keep you feeling full much longer than the higher-glycemic index carbohydrates

After the First Six Weeks

If you reach a plateau after the first six weeks, check several things.

- Check the label and see how many carbohydrates and how much sugar your food contains. Certain foods will slow down and even STOP weight loss. Foods with sugar or high-glycemic carbohydrates, including things you may not think about like fruits, fruit juices, condiments, potatoes, soft drinks, breads, and pastas.

- If you need a snack, make certain the snack is high in protein and not in carbohydrates or sugars. Snacking will slow down weight loss. A few extra bites of something contain calories you do not need.

- Do not skip meals. Meals are planned for, so it is easy to have nutritious food that has fewer calories (and lower glycemic index carbohydrates). If you skip meals, you will feel more like eating snacks, and snacks are filled with lots of dense calories. Skipping meals does not help to lose weight. In fact, the more you skip meals, the longer it takes for you to get to your goal weight (a BMI of 22).

- Remember to eat three meals a day, not three hundred. Grazing will kill your diet. You can slowly consume a lot of calories by grazing. If a meal is taking longer than 30 minutes to finish, you are grazing. The first few weeks you should eat a little bit at a time, but then you need to transition into three meals a day. This transition is difficult because you cannot believe that a two-inch square of salmon will fill you.

- Exercise. If you are not walking, the world is passing you by. Walk, walk, walk, and walk. When you are tired of walking, walk again. There is no excuse. If you need a new hip, knee, back, or other joint, then get involved in water aerobics. My favorite excuse is, "I walk a lot at work." More about walking later. Essentially, if you are not dedicating some time to exercise, you are missing the boat. I suggest you purchase a recumbent bike.

- Count carbohydrates. The more carbohydrates you consume, the harder it is to lose weight. Sixty grams a day should be MORE than enough. Check the carbohydrates you are eating and see where they fit on the glycemic index scale. There is also a list of common glycemic index carbohydrates on my website http://www.drsimpson.com.

- Check the sugar content. Natural sugar and honey are still sugar and natural fruits contain sugar. Your body really doesn't care if little elves, an organic mistress, or mom made the cake you eat. Just because it is natural does not mean your body won't grab the calories. Believe me, your body loves sugar, and it will grab onto every molecule and hang onto it for dear life. If you don't believe me, you are not my patient.

- Check the calendar. For women, your menstrual cycle will affect your weight. During certain times of the month, you will retain more fluid and weigh more. There is a natural urge to snack more during these times. That is why you should keep a supply of sugar-free fudgesickles—darn it!

- Skip the Happy Hour. Alcohol contains calories. Wine and beer have a lot of carbohydrates and alcohol has a lot of calories per serving. After surgery you will absorb alcohol quickly (you will become a cheap date).

How To Get Off the Plateau

—and back into the loss column: six months and beyond

You have two choices: cut calories (and the most common source of these are with high-glycemic index carbohydrates) or start walking. I love it when patients tell me they are going to the gym. Going to the gym does not mean exercise. Years ago, I went to a workout room at a hotel where I was staying. A woman came there dressed in appropriate workout clothes and walked around the room as if she were a priestess blessing the machines. There was no "work out." She spent maybe five minutes on one exercise bike, but she could now tell the world she went to the "fitness center" at the hotel.

Your body is a perfect calorie counter. It will measure what you take in and what goes out. You cannot fool it. Your body is not impressed that you took it to a gym. However, if you are stuck on a plateau, you need to work your way off of it. Just 45 minutes of sweating will do it. Watching a tape of some little ugly man swishing with old ladies does not cause you to lose weight.

You now have a tool that you never had before and dieting is a lot more successful because of this tool. Dieting before surgery didn't work well, but it will now. It will work for one simple reason—you cannot eat as much as you used to. If you once had a 50-ounce stomach and now have a one-ounce stomach, you will be satisfied with a lot less. Even after a year or two, we see pouches stretch to ten ounces without the person regaining weight.

Before surgery, you had to eat a garden full of vegetables and half a cow in order to fill full. Now it takes a few ounces of tuna fish to satisfy you. The smaller stomach allows you to feel full with less, so you don't have the urge to consume large quantities of food. The way to lose is not to stop eating; it is to make healthier choices. You now have a tool that you dreamed about before surgery. Remember your skinny sister-in-law who preaches about self-discipline? Well, your body can now enjoy a discipline it couldn't before, so make the choices.

Our goal is not just to get you to a BMI of 22, although that should be your goal and you can reach it. Those great before and after pictures you have seen, well—those are very dedicated patients. Their success was not the result of a specific surgery or surgeon; it was the result of a disciplined patient. Dieting may not have worked too well for you before the surgery, but after the surgery, dieting will work a lot better.

So, limit the carbohydrates to those that have a lower-glycemic index, and start walking. You will get off the plateau, you will lose weight, and you will be surprised how easily you can do this.

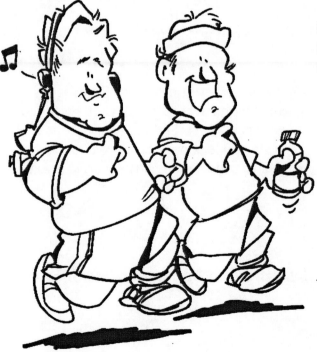

Finally—when thinking of the plateaus that you might be on, remember the commandments.

Dr. Simpson's Ten Commandments

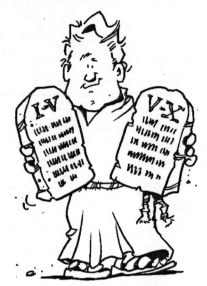

(1) Thou shalt learn the size of thy stomach and not overfill it.

(2) Thou shalt eat protein first.

(3) Thou shalt sip, not gulp thy liquids.

(4) Thou shalt walk every day.

(5) Thou shalt not smoke.

(6) Thou shalt chew thy food.

(7) Thou shalt take thy vitamins and supplements daily.

(8) Thou shalt not covet thy neighbors or thy child's plate.

(9) Thou shalt limit snacks to two a day, and plan them

(10) Thou shalt not graze.

Above all, weight loss surgery should not ever make your life miserable. It is simply a tool. There is nothing wrong with having some dessert, but if you are on a plateau and have not reached your goal, you might consider putting it aside for a little bit or walking it off later. Our goal is to provide you with a tool that will make a diet work well for you and help you get out of the morbid obesity category.

Your Mantra

There are no bad foods; there are only bad quantities of foods.

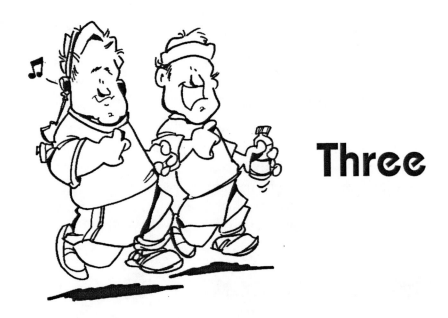

Three

Exercise

–is not a four-letter word

Exercise is something that you know is healthy, something you feel you should do, but it is difficult to consider exercise when you have a lot of excess weight. Now that you have had surgery (or are thinking about surgery, and reading ahead), it is time to begin an exercise program. No, really—don't turn the page—this is serious. I say this as I return from a two-mile walk feeling great. I'm also sweating hard and wondering if help will arrive here in time if I dial 911.

Walking is the simplest of all exercises. Walking around your office at work during the day does not count. That's what you do for a living. Exercise is time you dedicate to doing something just for yourself. One of my favorite lines from Jimmy Buffet is, *Your body is a temple, don't treat it like a tent* (paraphrased, but in the audio edition of this book I will sing it).

No excuses are accepted here. Besides, there are a lot of benefits. The time you are walking provides you free time to think, your weight loss to proceed much faster, helps your bowels move better, and gives you an overall feeling of good health. Okay, initially you won't always feel so great. In fact, the worst part of exercise is thinking about it. Once you do it, you actually feel better.

The goal is to increase walking until you are walking four miles in one hour and doing that four times a week. This is not a leisurely walk, this is a paced program, a fast walk. You should strive for this goal before surgery and plan to get back to it as soon as you can after surgery. If you are now a few months post-operative and you are still not back to exercising, it is time to think about it. All right, now that you have thought about it—how do you start?

Before You Start...

First, talk to your doctor. Not just your surgeon, but also your primary care doctor or your cardiologist. Do not start without doing this. Your doctor, or the nurse, will also show you how to take your own pulse because during this time you will need to monitor your pulse rate. Your doctor may even have some target goals for you. You will want to check your pulse because, as you become more conditioned, your pulse rate will decrease.

Your heart rate should not exceed 220 minus your age in years, so, if you are 40 years old, your maximum heart rate should be 180 beats per minute. We want your heart rate to reach about 60 to 80 percent of the maximum. (For example, if you are 40 years old, then your heart rate should be 110 to 140 beats per minute). You should go over this with your doctor because some people will require different goals and some medicines will affect the heart rate (beta blockers like propranolol). You should also visit a physical therapist. He will not only help you get started on a program, but can show you some simple things to do to prevent injury. The best time to prevent injury is before your walk—by stretching properly, and after your walk during the cooling down phase.

When I started to jog (which was a long time ago) I was told that if I couldn't talk while I was jogging, then I probably needed a rest. The same is true with walking. If you cannot talk, then you need to rest and catch your breath. But for me, not talking is difficult no matter what I am doing so I knew that if I couldn't talk, then something was wrong.

During your walk, check your pulse. If you have one of those gizmos that do it for you, great, but you do need to learn to check your own (in case the batteries in your gizmo die).

The next part is also easy for most people: you have to go shopping. Yup, if you are going to start this program, reward yourself by purchasing the right stuff for your walk. Start with a good pair of walking shoes. Almost any foot store or athletic foot store will help you with this. Shoes are critical. You want a pair of shoes that supports you and fits well. Clothing for walking is also important. I highly recommend cotton (Pima cotton, of course). Select clothes that breathe, are easy to clean, and are stylish. So, shop for shoes, some t-shirts, a nice pair of walking shorts, and go for it.

Shoes are critical. You want a pair of shoes that supports you and fits well.

If you want to spend some real money, get a pedometer, a device that tells you how far you have walked. They cost about twenty bucks. If you have the cash, you might even get one of those little devices that tell you your heart rate (some watches have them).

Living in Phoenix means I have heard the "it is too hot" excuse from many patients. When I lived in Alaska, the excuse was "the weather is too bad," or "it's raining too much." The only acceptable excuse for skipping your exercise is one from your physician. The key is to find a fun place to walk. Shopping malls are fun because they are air conditioned and you can window shop for new clothes as your sizes change. Walking is just that, it is walking—it isn't wandering, it isn't a slow saunter, it is walking at a nice brisk pace.

Next, you need a walking buddy. If you have someone to go with you, it helps motivate you on days when you just don't want to do it. In fact, it is best to get a few of you together to walk. The more the merrier. If you can't find a human, get a dog. They love to walk and will insist on going at least once every day.

The Walking Program

The first time you walk, make it one quarter of a mile. And again, you should be walking with a friend and you should have checked with your doctor. Most cities are built with eight blocks to the mile, so this would be one block out, and one block back.

Walk one quarter of a mile the first day, rest a day, then two days of walking a quarter of a mile, followed by a day off. Essentially your walking prescription will be walk one day, rest one day, walk two days, rest one day, and repeat. After a week of doing this, you need to increase by a quarter of a mile. This may not seem like much, but remember our goal, ten weeks after you start this program is to get you to walk four miles a day, four times a week, and to walk it in just under an hour.

Week	Mon.	Tues.	Wed.	Thurs.	Fri.	Sat.	Sun.
1	1/4 mile	Rest	1/4 mile	1/4 mile	Rest	1/4 mile	1/2 mile
2	Rest	1/2 mile	Rest	1/2 mile	1/2 mile	Rest	3/4 mile
3	3/4 mile	Rest	3/4 mile	Rest	3/4 mile	1 mile	rest

There—you can fill in the rest. You get the idea—a nice easy weekly pace.

There are a few things you need to do first. First, check with your doctor, learn how to check your pulse or get a pulse-checking gizmo. Next, after you have walked half way, check your pulse. If you have not reached your target, then you need to pick up the pace. Check your pulse again when you have completed your walk (sometimes you will need to check it more often, but again, consult with your doctor). Ten minutes after you have finished your walk, your heart rate should have decreased and you should be able to catch your breath.

Warm Up and Cool Down

Before you start your walk, you need to stretch. Here is where the physical therapist can help you with some simple stretching and breathing exercises. You need to get warmed up just a bit before you go marching off through the mall. When you are finished walking, you need to cool down a bit. Don't just plop in a chair and looked dazed. Cool down by slowing down to a gentle walk. Go check out the men's clothing store to buy a Dr. Simpson t-shirt. Warm up—cool down.

Contact your physician if you notice any of the following:

(a) chest pain after or during exercise. This might indicate some heart trouble.

(b) light-headedness

(c) heart rate which decreases during exercise

(d) joint pain

But Doctor, My Joints Hurt

Doing water aerobics is a great way to exercise and is gentle on the joints. An exercise bike is great. You can put it in your living room or den (or wherever you want to put it), where it doesn't rain or get too hot. I had a Nordic-trac once; it was a great place to hang clothes. The key to using a piece of exercise equipment is to exercise with a buddy or a group. So, instead of spending the money on some home equipment, join a gym. If you live near a city, go to the mall and walk. Many malls open a couple of hours before the stores do just so people can walk and exercise. Also, you will meet a lot of interesting people there getting their laps in before the stores open. There is always some place to exercise.

If you cannot exercise, then you probably cannot, or should not, have surgery. There are some notable exceptions to this, but again, if your doctor gives you an excuse to skip the exercise, then share it with your surgeon. It will help him or her decide if you really are a good candidate for surgery or not, and if so, which type of surgery you should have. Surgery creates major stress on your body, more so than any walking or exercise program. If you cannot take the stress of walking or some other exercise, then you cannot, or should not, have surgery.

What You Should Expect from Exercise

(a) Your heart rate should increase during the exercise and then return to normal within ten minutes.

(b) You should feel some fatigue and soreness in your muscles, which will improve over the next day or two.

(c) You should feel a sense of "accomplishment" or improvement as the weeks go by.

Exercise will make you feel better. Many patients find that once they start exercising, they enjoy doing it and they enjoy the results. You will find that your clothes fit better, and you have more stamina to do things you enjoy (yes, those things too). One of my good friends who had this surgery done now calls himself a gym-rat. He is not only enjoying the benefits of weight loss surgery, but feels that exercise is sculpting his body.

Let us be honest: most of you will hate the thought of exercise but like the idea of what it can do for you. It is easy to become discouraged, to quit, and yet this is one of the best things you can do. How do I know this? Beause I hate to walk. I mean, I like the feeling of accomplishment but if it were not for my buddy dragging my fat belly out the door I would be peacefully sitting in front of my computer surfing the internet. So, get a buddy, check with your doctor, purchase some stuff, and go for it!

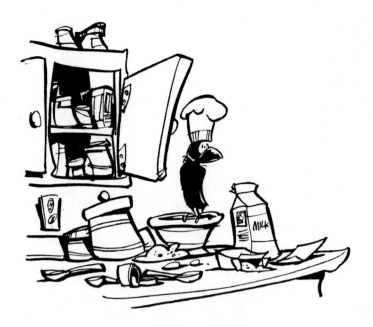

Four

Your Post-Op Diet

What to Eat the First 12 Weeks

Your first diet after surgery will be clear liquids. A diet of clear liquids maintains vital body fluids, salts, and minerals; and also gives you some energy until you can resume a normal diet. Clear liquids are easily absorbed by the body. This eases the digestive tract into processing food again after the trauma of surgery.

What is a clear liquid? A good rule-of-thumb is anything you can see through. For example, apple juice is a clear liquid; milk is not. If unsure, check with the physician or registered dietitian. Clear liquids are any transparent drinkable liquid. Like glass, it might have color but you should still be able to see through it. Usually they contain mostly water and sugar (or sugar substitute, except for broths and bullion, which are salty). A strict clear liquid diet excludes all solids (even noodles in soup), milk products, and citrus (orange or grapefruit) juices. See Appendix One for examples.

Liquid Diets

Honestly, your surgeon is not torturing you

Some surgeons have their patients stay on liquid diets for several weeks after surgery. Some surgeons allow patients to eat solids fairly early on. Everyone seems to have a different plan. Who is right? Your surgeon is. Follow his plan because he has a very specific reasons for the diet he gives you.

Liquids empty from the stomach, or the pouch, differently than solids. You can survive with just liquids for a long time. The rationale for liquids is that they won't stretch the pouch—unless you gulp them. So, sip, sip, and sip.

There are two variations of liquid diets: clear liquids and full liquids. The appendix shows you the difference. The real question is not what is a liquid; the

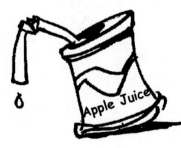

real question is what is coffee. Okay, so I fudge a little bit here, but I do this because of Ira. Ira's only request was that he be allowed to drink coffee when he left the recovery room. I made a deal that we would call coffee a clear liquid if he would do laps around the nurse's station. Ira became the world-marathon hospital lapper and he had his coffee. Now 100-plus pounds later, Ira is a fixture in our support group and a great encouragement to others—and we love talking about our favorite restaurants (yup, Peter Lugar Steak House in the Big Apple or Cafe Sport in San Francisco).

Most surgeons who have patients on prolonged liquid diets are concerned about the staple line leaking. They want to give the stomach a chance to heal and liquids do pass through the stomach quickly. Also, a liquid diet helps you to lose weight.

The key to healing is getting in enough protein. There are many varieties of protein drinks available. There are also a lot of recipes for putting tofu in a blender with various things and making great shakes. Unfortunately a lot of "smoothies" are very high in carbohydrates and not terribly appropriate for weight loss.

Clear Liquids

Controversies with clear liquids

Diabetic patients show no significant increase in blood sugar when they are started on a clear liquid diet containing sugar following surgery.

The Puree Diet

No, you cannot puree a Big Mac

A blender is important during this phase, as it allows food items to be pureed to the consistency of baby food, yogurt, or applesauce. See Appendix One.

The puree, or blender diet, is meant to allow patients with a limited capacity to have foods that go down easily without stretching the pouch, or stomach. The puree diet limits the post-operative vomiting that patients might have, and vomiting is the enemy. Vomiting leads to increased incidence of leaks, breakdown of the staple line, and band slips. A puree diet increases the diversity of food that you can eat and increases protein sources. During this time, a chewable vitamin should be taken.

TIP: A coffee bean grinder works well to grind up pills

Once the pills are ground place them in a teaspoon, add some Splenda® and a drop of water. Swallow the medicine and follow it with some water. You can also place the medicine in some applesauce and take it that way.

Consume Six Small Meals Per Day

You will transition to three meals per day and a snack, but during this period, it is important to begin regulating your food. Until the first 12 weeks are done, and your surgeon agrees, do not eat and drink at the same time. We let patients sip with their food after six weeks and have found no problem with this.

Your Pouch Size

Measure Twice, Eat Once

So, measure everything you eat. If it is more than your stomach size, DO NOT CHANCE IT. Better to eat less and not vomit than to eat more and purge yourself. Vomiting is not a fun way to lose weight. You will lose weight if you eat too much and vomit, but it is uncomfortable, and at the most it can cause severe problems including electrolyte imbalance, tearing your stomach or esophagus, or ripping staple lines. You can prevent most vomiting by watching and measuring what you eat. In time you will be able to "eyeball" your food and determine how much you should eat.

Measuring your food seems silly, but it is not. One of the great items to have on hand is a shot glass: it can be your best friend in times of trouble. Okay—so you want to hear a story about a shot glass. This is also a story about measuring. John is a great friend of mine, a bright fellow with two master's degrees who started out life as a plumber. John's favorite job was owner of a bar; in fact John is looking to purchase a bar again (Seattle bar owners, feel free to apply). John told me that there are "professional" drinkers. Some of these would come to his bar and ask for a shot of their favorite beverage (whiskey for my dad, vodka for my friend Chuck, and for me, tequila. They would throw the shot into their mouth, and they would measure the shot with their mouth. If it was five-eighths of an ounce they got up and left the bar. If it was a full ounce or more, he had a new, steady customer. The point is (yes, you were probably wondering) that you should learn to measure your food but, unlike our barflies, we want you to swallow it slowly. If you eat slowly you will not experience discomfort and you will know what it feels like to be full.

A weighty issue well-measured

Boerhaave syndrome is a rupture of the esophagus after forceful vomiting. This syndrome is named after the surgeon who described a Dutch admiral who overate, vomited, ruptured his esophagus, and the contents of his stomach were found in his chest (at autopsy). This can easily happen to post-operative patients who overfill their small stomach (or pouch). It is fatal if not treated early. Two weeks after her duodenal switch, a patient of mine overate, vomited, and ruptured her esophagus. After chest surgery, a few days in the ICU, and a month in the hospital, she finally went home. Measure twice, eat once, and vomit never! This is also a reason you should *NEVER* induce vomiting.

The question is, how much does your stomach hold?

Ounces	Milliliters	Cups	Tablespoons
1 ounce	30 cc	1/8 cup	2 tablespoons
4 ounces	120 cc	1/2 cup	8 tablespoons
8 ounces	240 cc	1 cup	16 tablespoons
40 ounces	1.2 liters	5 cups	80 tablespoons
50 ounces	1.5 liters	6.25 cups	100 tablespoons

It is astounding to think that the average stomach holds between 40 and 50 ounces before weight loss surgery. When you compare the before and after size of the stomach, it is clear why patients are amazed at how full they feel with so much less food.

I hate to bring up vomiting again (by now you must be used to my puns). When you have a regular stomach and you vomit, you might put a bit of beverage in it to help calm it down. When you have a one-ounce pouch or a 4-ounce stomach, putting a bit in is a lot! Would you eat a 10-ounce steak to calm down your stomach? Of course not! But having a "sip" of soda, or drinking some water can fill that one-ounce stomach up, stretching it and causing you to regurgitate its contents. This is why the first rule of an upset stomach is to STOP, relax, and once your stomach settles down, go back to the clear liquids as prescribed.

How much weight can you lose with such a small stomach/pouch?

During my Friday afternoon chats one of the common questions is, "How will my body know when to stop losing weight?" The implication is that post-operative patients will lose so much weight they will dry up and blow away. This doesn't happen. The stomach remnant will expand a bit over time so you will be able to hold more food. Every now and then we hear of someone who loses too much weight after surgery, and these unfortunate individuals may have other problems. In fact, the problem most patients face is not losing too much, but getting rid of the last 30-50 pounds.

Honestly, two tablespoons are enough

Well-meaning friends and family will be concerned that you are not getting enough to eat—you are. These same individuals may think you are losing too much weight too fast, and sometimes even a physician will tell patients that they shouldn't be losing so much weight.

With some very notable exceptions (for example, you are rapidly approaching a BMI of 18 and not reaching a plateau) weight loss is expected to be very rapid, especially early on. Do not force yourself to eat more; if you force yourself to eat what others think you should, you may stretch your stomach. If you are 100-pounds overweight, your body contains enough calories to sustain yourself for six months with just fluids and some supplements.

Discipline is something people use in a negative sense. Every person who has a few pounds to lose has heard that term used, as in, "If only you had some discipline you would have never gotten this way," In case you didn't know, "this way" is their politically-correct euphemism for "fat." However, after weight loss surgery, your body enforces a discipline that is beyond the "will." Your body's "discipline" is a complex mechanism of appetite and feeling full. In this case, because of your new anatomy, your "discipline" has changed substantially from what it was before surgery. So learn it, test it, feel it, but most important, measure it.

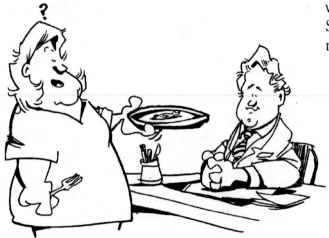

Appetites and Feeling Full

Appetite, and feeling full are complex interactions that occur somewhere in the brain, and are based on signals from the stomach. There is a disease, Prader-Willi syndrome, where the brain does not recognize satiety (the feeling of being full). These unfortunate individuals become morbidly obese as they have no internal mechanism to tell them when they should feel full, and they always feel hungry. In simple terms, when your stomach begins to feel full it sends a signal to the brain which says, "Hey, I am full here so don't throw anything more down or I will throw it back up." That is the feeling I have after a Thanksgiving Dinner—usually after I have had seconds and have just finished off a nice pumpkin pie. But this feeling doesn't happen the instant that the stomach is stretched. This sensation takes a while to reach the brain. The signal may be from the hormone ghrelin. This hormone is found in low levels in patients who have had the Roux-en-Y gastric bypass and in patients who are obese. Sounds strange? When obese patients who begin to diet the level goes up, stimulating the appetite. The levels are low because they are constantly eating and keeping the level low.

Many obese patients have an aberration in their satiety mechanism. They don't know when they are full. It is something they have not experienced. These early 12 weeks are a great time to get in touch with that feeling. Measure your food, eat your food, and know what satiety feels like. If you have had Roux-en-Y gastric bypass surgery and you are tolerating chicken, measure out an ounce of chicken (assuming you have a one-ounce pouch) and SLOWLY eat it. Wait a bit and notice that feeling you have; your stomach's upper pouch is full and your stomach is signaling your brain that you don't need to eat any more. Again, some days you cannot eat one ounce, only a tablespoon will do. That is okay.

Phantom Hunger Pains

Did you ever hear of a person who had an amputation and complained that his toes hurt? Phantom pain is a well-known phenomenon in medicine, and it applies to more than just feet. Some days you will feel hungry even though you are filled. There are a lot of complex theories as to why this occurs. It is real, but we are going to tell you about a few tricks to make it better.

One trick is water loading. Because of a limited stomach capacity, you learn to eat and not to drink at the same time. This doesn't change. Don't start eating and drinking together but you *can* start to drink more between meals. Two hours after eating, begin drinking a lot of water. The water will fill you up, it doesn't have any calories, and while the feeling of being full won't last long, it provides a few minutes of relief when you would otherwise reach for something that has a lot of calories. Water loading isn't something you can hope to remember, it is something to plan for. If you find that you snack every day at a certain time, try drinking water before that time and you will have a less intense hunger. It will relieve the phantom hunger pain and allow you to continue to lose weight.

Protein Drinks, Shakes, Bars and Other "Foods"

—or, sawdust in a bottle

I admit that I don't like the taste of most protein drinks, shakes or bars. I prefer that patients meet their protein requirements with food such as fish, poultry, tofu, cheese, egg whites. However, there are a number of patients who have such a difficult time with food the first few weeks that these alternative sources of protein seem to work well. Whey-based protein products or egg-white based products generally have more "bioavailability" than soy products. This means that more of the protein can be absorbed and used by the body. See Appendix One for protein requirements.

After surgery is a great time to try new sources of protein, especially fish (sushi) or tofu. Tofu is a "high-quality" protein, a protein that is low in fat. There are several vegetarian restaurants in Phoenix that have excellent tofu meals, and these are quite easily tolerated in the early post-operative period. I am not a vegetarian; in fact I believe taking baby carrots from their mothers is cruel and unusual. Tofu and soy-based products, such as "Morning Star" brands, are available in supermarkets. No longer do you need to go to a health food store to purchase soy-based products.

Lactose Intolerance

It is common problem, so how do we get calcium?

Foods that contain lactose:

- milk
- cream
- ice Cream
- cheese
- many sauces, soups, salad dressings, and prepared foods (check the labels for "lactose")
- some prescription drugs and medicines

It is very common after any surgery on the gut for patients to develop what we call "lactose intolerance." Lactose is "milk sugar" and is broken down by enzymes in the gut. After surgery these enzymes (called lactase) may take a vacation and may not come back.

Lactose intolerance is common among many people. Symptoms are cramps, bloating, diarrhea, nausea, lots of gas, and a noisy gut. The undigested milk sugar (lactose) becomes food for bacteria that live in the colon. The bacteria break down the lactose and you start to feel the symptoms. Usually symptoms occur thirty minutes to two hours after you have the lactose-containing foods.

You can purchase "lactase" tablets, or milk that has had much of the lactose removed or broken down. This is something you will have to experiment with. Some patients have such problems with lactose intolerance that the slightest bit of milk sugar will cause them to have severe cramping and pain in the stomach. Other patients find they can eat yogurt, cottage cheese, and hard cheeses, but cannot tolerate milk or ice cream. Yogurt is very low in lactose.

Lactose intolerance is common among Native Americans. When I worked at the Indian Hospital and patients became constipated they would drink a glass of milk to relieve the constipation. Being one-quarter Native American and one-half Norwegian, my body doesn't know what it is supposed to do with milk. However, I find I can get by just fine if I don't drink milk and if I limit my ice cream to four scoops!

Calcium is present in high quantities in all dairy foods but these also contain lactose. If you are lactose-intolerant you should supplement your diet with calcium. Some vegetables have a lot of calcium such as kale, collard greens, broccoli, and turnip greens. I prefer to take Tums®.

Gluten Intolerance

Celiac Disease

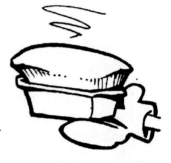

Celiac disease is caused by an allergy to gluten. Gluten is a substance found in wheat, barley, and rye. It can be difficult to diagnose Celiac disease even though it causes multiple symptoms. Patients can suffer from diarrhea, weight loss, and nutritional deficiencies (making it difficult to differentiate from a lot of other things that post-operative patients develop). This is a disease that can become unmasked by the surgery. Treatment is important because if patients continue to eat a diet with gluten they often have a 40-times higher risk of developing gastrointestinal cancer than anyone else.

Perhaps the most famous patient with this is an author of cookbooks. She was such a good cook that she weighed 185 pounds more than she should have. She had successful Roux-en-Y bypass, done by a good friend of mine, and did spectacularly well. She was religious in her avoidance of high-glycemic index carbohydrates (which also happen to contain gluten). She was full of energy and did a lot of traveling. She slowly reintroduced carbohydrates into her diet, always watching her scale to make certain she maintained her weight around 130 pounds, and then became chronically ill.

She suffered from severe diarrhea, bloating, and intestinal pain. She was hospitalized several times and even had her gallbladder out, which everyone thought would cure her. However, she continued to become weaker and weaker. After passing out a few times from dehydration, she decided to seek specialized medical attention. Multiple endoscopies were performed, one of which showed she had severe bile-salt diarrhea (which they thought was a consequence of having her gallbladder removed).

Every time she ate, she became sick. Her diarrhea was so bad she was confined to her home, and the odor from the gas was so bad that she refused to travel except for short distances to the store. She was given multiple diagnoses, including irritable bowel syndrome, post-cholecystectomy syndrome, bacterial overgrowth, and bile-salt diarrhea. Finally, she became so ill that the physicians decided to place her on total bowel rest by placing a special intravenous line in her that fed her with Total Parentral Nutrition (TPN).

Within a week she was feeling energetic again, and within two weeks she was feeling even better. It took almost two months of total intravenous nutrition to get her back to normal. The support system of post-operative patients is world-wide and she had, through the internet, discussed her situation with some close friends, one of whom happened to be a physician. He suggested Celiac disease might be the problem and told her to watch what happened when she ate products with gluten. Being an internet-savvy individual, she looked up every website and learned as much as she could about the disease.

A Gluten-Free Diet Worked

Her primary care physician checked her blood for the disease but it was negative (which was, by the way, entirely expected as she had been off all food for several weeks). She ate a pretzel with peanut butter and cramped for a day. She then discovered a store nearby that specialized in gluten-free products and is probably now rewriting a cookbook with her famous recipes made gluten-free.

This young woman nearly died, as some do, but now is back to her usual spunky self and no doubt will be America's replacement for Julia Child (but if she has a television program you can bet, the food she puts in her mouth will be gluten-free). In reading about some patients who have become progressively malnourished and died following weight loss surgery, I cannot help but wonder if they are included in the one-in-133 people who have Celiac disease unmasked by the surgery.

Carbohydrates

–Top or Bottom of the Pyramid?

No weight loss surgery will inhibit the absorption of carbohydrates and sugar. If you do not limit the total amount of carbohydrates (and sugar) you consume you will lose the effect of this surgery. Carbohydrates are simply long chains of sugars strung together that your body will break down and absorb. Nutrition and the famous food pyramid are about as interesting as watching corn grow. It seems you should be able to simply eat and all the proteins, minerals, vitamins, and other stuff would take care of themselves. Who really has time to figure out if they are eating portions of fruit, dairy, or vegetables anyway?

Even when I was a kid and everything was interesting, the food pyramid seemed like a rip off. I mean, the real pyramids in Egypt, now they were interesting. Then I became a bariatric surgeon, and guess what—it is still boring! So, forget the food pyramid, they are reworking it anyway and no doubt will be different. In the traditional food pyramid, carbohydrates were the building block upon which all other food groups rested. If we were to build a pyramid for weight loss surgery patients, we would want protein to be at the base, or the foundation for all meals. That is why we have meal plans and menus at the end of this book.

There Are No Bad Foods

–but there are bad quantities of them

Sometimes talking about certain foods to patients who have reached their goal weight is like talking to an alcoholic about vodka. Some patients who reached their goal had a simple, single vision of where they wanted to go, identified those foods that got them in trouble, and avoided them zealously. Most who reached their goal avoided highly processed, high-glycemic index carbohydrates—potatoes, bread, rice, and pasta (although there are some pastas that have a lower-glycemic index, these pastas are not the ones typically found in restaurants). They also avoided fast food places, with specific exceptions. Once they were within sight of their goal, they expanded their diet but were wary of certain foods and watched the scale.

Those are the two simple approaches: complete avoidance of the high-carbohydrate foods that commonly cause obesity, or a rational reintroduction of certain carbohydrates into your diet according to your BMI. If you find that you only eat those foods that cause obesity such as, high-glycemic carbohydrates (sugars, candy, soda, potatoes, breads), fats (red meat, butter, cream, hamburgers) or common combinations of the two (donuts, ice cream, potatoes with butter and sour cream), then you must change your eating habits. Why change? Besides obesity, a diet that contains a lot of calories generally does not contain a lot of nutrition. So, while you may succeed in having plenty of calories, you may become progressively malnourished and fat. After any weight loss surgery, there is a limited amount of food you can take in. Because of that enforced limitation, if you do not eat properly you will not do well. This means, sigh, you must learn what you need to eat. You probably need to learn some new recipes, and when you eat out make certain you are eating foods that have a high nutritional value.

High-Glycemic Carbohydrates

—or, the carbs that don't stick to your ribs, only to your thighs

Not all carbohydrates are created equal. (See Appendix One.) Some carbohydrates cause an immediate rise in blood sugar, peaking quickly then falling, leaving you hungry faster. These carbohydrates have a high-glycemic index. Examples of these are breads, potatoes, sugar, and candy. Other carbohydrates cause a much slower rise in blood sugar and give you the sensation of feeling full for hours after eating them. These carbohydrates have a low-glycemic index. Examples of these include apples, lentils, beans, and most vegetables.

I love the Atkins diet because I am a meat eater by nature and never hesitate to have half a heifer for dinner. Having a breakfast of steak and eggs makes me feel rich and full. The Atkins diet has a low-carbohydrate approach to life, and the simple counting of carbohydrates makes the diet easy to follow and quite successful. But, all carbohydrates are not created equal.

This is where the glycemic index comes in. All carbohydrates are not equal at all. Take my morning choice. When I go to the surgery lounge at the hospital, they have a wonderful selection of donuts and fruit. Now an apple contains about

25 grams of carbohydrate, and a donut contains the same. So which is better? Okay, the apple is better, but why? If we are just talking about carbohydrates, then 25 grams is 25 grams, isn't it? The answer is no, because the glycemic index is different. A donut has a glycemic index of around 75, which is fairly high. This means you will eat the donut and you will have a rapid rise in blood sugar, which will peak and then decrease rapidly, leaving you feeling hungry. An apple has a glycemic index of 34, which is fairly low. The apple will cause a slow rise in blood sugar, and you will maintain that low level for several hours. You won't get the quick rise or quick fall and you will feel full longer. But even more, the apple contains more vitamins, better nutrition, and more fiber than the donut. Okay, you probably knew that, but we just gave the scientific reason.

High-glycemic foods tend to cause obesity, diabetes, heart disease, and even cancer. Does that mean you must never have that donut, the white bread, or the lasagna? Not at all, the good news is that if you combine a low-glycemic food with a high-glycemic food you average the load. Eat those vegetables! At one time if you were diagnosed with diabetes, you were told you could never have sugar again; now the thinking is that we should eat a combination of foods to decrease the glycemic index as much as possible.

How can you tell the high-glycemic foods from the low-glycemic ones? There is no simple answer. There is no test to tell us which is a high or low-glycemic food, we simply must test the food by feeding a specified quantity to people and watching for the blood sugar response to all this. In the not so distant past we thought that "complex carbohydrate" was the same as a low-glycemic food, but those notions have gone the way of the buggy whip. For a while we assumed that fiber in the carbohydrates would slow digestion. Fiber does help a great deal in foods, but fiber isn't the only answer. These are still reports disputing this in the popular press, but for this year, glycemic index, determined through testing, is our best approximation of how your body will react to certain foods.

Counting Carbs, Not Crows

There are two approaches to carbohydrates, one is to simply count them and not exceed a certain number. This works well in the early stages following weight loss surgery but not always later on. (See Appendix One.)

For carbohydrate-counters, the total daily amount of carbohydrates should not exceed 60 grams, or 20 grams of carbohydrates per meal. If you consume more than this amount, you risk regaining weight. Remember, carbohydrates and sugars are not your friend. Sugar is in many things that you might not even consider: fruit juices, processed food products, condiments such as ketchup, and also in canned fruits, pastry products, pasta, breads, and even some vegetables. Sugar is very well absorbed after this surgery, so the more sugars and carbohydrates you eat, the longer it will take to lose weight.

Snacks cause most people to stop losing weight or to lose it slower. Many snacks are high in carbohydrates and low in protein. Your goal is to find snacks that are higher in protein than carbohydrates. Some protein bars make good snacks, but some contain far more carbohydrates than we would like to see you consume. Shrimp is a good single-bite snack with protein. Nuts and seeds are fairly high in protein. We have a few snack suggestions in the menu section. This is where you should become a label watcher.

Glycemic Index and BMI

Which carbohydrates should I re-introduce?

Another successful approach is matching the foods that you eat with your BMI. The rule is simple: If your BMI is over 35 have foods with a glycemic index no greater than 55. For a BMI between 25 and 35, have foods with a glycemic index no greater than 70. Once your BMI is below 25, there is no restriction on foods you can have. Simply have protein first.

I advocate this approach for patients once they are past their first 12 weeks. It is fairly easy to follow. Of course here I can shamelessly promote my book that has a carbohydrate counter and glycemic index table all in one, but I will resist that urge.

Exceptions to the Rules

There are no exceptions unless you are one of those patients who has a severe need for carbohydrates because of exercise. However, one of my patients even gained weight training for a marathon! If you think you are an exception, you will have to prove yourself. You do not need a Snickers bar for walking, running, or playing tennis. If you feel you need to "load" carbohydrates, remember you need to sustain the release of glucose over time. This means you cannot load with high-glycemic foods. If you want to load, then load with low-glycemic items so glucose will be released slowly over a period of time.

Restaurants and Eating at Your In-laws

At restaurants you will find that appetizers are often the perfect portion size for your stomach and they contain good food. Smoked salmon, shrimp cocktail, oysters—are all good sources of protein. Ask for the appetizer instead of the main dish. If you really want the main dish, then once you get your food, ask for a take-home box. Divide your food into portions and put the rest in a box. A nice 6-ounce fillet might make two or three meals. It is best to portion it out first. If you are tempted to eat more than you should, remember that restaurant restrooms are not as comfortable as yours at home.

When visiting friends or in-laws who may not know—and do not need to know—that you have had weight loss surgery, tell them ahead of time that you need smaller portions. Tell them you have had stomach surgery (they don't need to know what kind) and that they can all understand what it means. You can tell them that you need high-protein foods.

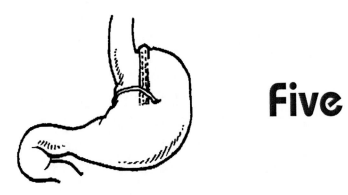

Five

Tips for VBG Patients

The key to an easy recovery period after VBG surgery is to avoid overfilling the pouch and avoid vomiting, especially the first few days. There is one way to do this: measure twice, swallow once, and vomit never.

This surgery needs time to heal. Most surgeons require that you be on a pureed diet for the first six weeks after surgery. Remember, in this surgery the outlet is reinforced with a band (made of some plastic-type material) and cannot stretch. As with any surgery, some swelling happens immediately after surgery and this will make the pouch feel even tighter than normal.

A liquid diet for the first two weeks after surgery is normal and will allow the surgery to heal. The stoma (opening between the stomach sections) will swell a bit after surgery. This means if you cheat and have some food, it might get stuck. If food becomes stuck and serious vomiting occurs, you can disrupt the staple line, enlarge the pouch, and cause many problems. So, if your doctor wants you on a liquid diet, don't cheat.

Foods to Avoid the First Six Weeks

Avoid certain foods the first six weeks. These foods, if you eat them, will make you very uncomfortable. Some of them can get stuck in the stoma, and some will expand in the pouch and make you vomit. They might even rupture the staple line.

Foods that expand in the pouch and may make you uncomfortable:

- breads, pastas, granola. Go lightly on oatmeal.
- foods that can become stuck or cause bezoars (hair balls—here kitty)
- high-fiber vegetables (see Appendix One)
- pulp, cores, and seeds of fruits (avoid grapefruits, oranges, and bananas)

Rules of the VBG Pouch

This operation is designed to limit what you eat and make you feel full early. You can defeat the pouch, however. The way to defeat it is to drink when you eat, drink after you eat, or eat a lot of high-carbohydrate foods (milkshakes, French fries, candy, and the like).

The pouch is a tool, and the tool has to be used if you are going to reach your weight loss goal. As with any tool, there are some simple rules:

(a) The pouch is designed to be full with a limited amount of food. Once you feel full stop eating.

(b) The pouch is designed to keep you feeling full for a long period. You can defeat this by washing food out of the pouch so don't drink for an hour after you consume food. Now, this rule has been modified a bit. It seems that some liquid with meals works well and does not cause you to gain weight, but the key is to sip those liquids, not to gulp them or use the liquid to force down more food. The other key is to be very careful not to eat and drink at the same time during the first 12 weeks.

(c) If the pouch is empty, you can drink a lot of water or other liquids—but be smart—do not drink high-calorie liquids. Water is the best thing you can drink. Skim milk, unsweetened fruit juices, broth, coffee, or Crystal Lite® are good choices. Some surgeons feel that foods sweetened with Nutrasweet® products stimulate appetite. Some surgeons have absolute prohibitions against carbonation. You should SIP six to eight cups of fluid between meals. This will keep you hydrated.

(d) You should take a liquid or chewable multivitamin daily. If you are a pre-menstrual female, then you may need iron. Mineral supplements should be discussed with your surgeon or primary care doctor, depending upon your medical condition. Some surgeons state that because there is no "malabsorption" with this operation so are unnecessary. The National Academy of Science recommends that all Americans should have vitamin supplementation. (If you are not from America, do it anyway.)

(e) Chew your food, but before you put the food in your mouth, make certain that it is cut smaller than your little fingernail. (No, false nails cannot be used as a measurement device.) If you do not chew your food, you will be very sorry.

(f) Eat slowly. A meal should take between 15 and 30 minutes. Less than that means you are eating too fast, more than that means you are grazing.

(g) Eat three meals a day, and eat them at the same time each day.

(h) Purchase some smaller plates, forks, spoons, and use them for yourself and everyone else in the family. (Your family members will benefit from smaller portions. Honest, they will.)

(i) Food groups are meats, fruits, vegetables, and dairy. You should have a balanced meal with a bit from each category.

Items to eat the first few weeks:

- pureed meats
- cottage cheese (low-fat)
- pureed peaches
- pureed yams or sweet potatoes
- cooked, soft-grained cereal

After Three Months

The capacity of your pouch will increase over time. This is not unusual and is even expected. Typically, it will go from one ounce to four ounces. If it is larger than four ounces, this might indicate that the pouch has been overfed. You can do the cottage cheese test to see how large your pouch should be.

The Cottage Cheese Test

Get an unopened container of small-curd, low-fat cottage cheese. On an empty pouch, rapidly eat your fill. Measure the uneaten cottage cheese in the container, then deduct this measurement from the original container-size. For example: the original container held eight ounces of cottage cheese, and there is a four-ounce serving left. That means your pouch holds four ounces. This gives you the approximate functional size of your pouch. Sometimes cottage cheese goes through a pouch a bit too quickly, so tuna salad may work better for you.

Items to eat after three months:

After three months, you should strive for a well-balanced meal. While a wide range of foods is open to you, you must remember the rules of the VBG.

(a) Do not eat and drink at the same time. You can sip small amounts but do not use the liquid to force unchewed food into your stomach.

(b) Chew your food to a semi-solid (pudding) consistency

(c) Measure twice, eat once, and vomit never.

(d) Do not skip meals, and do not substitute snacks for a meal

(e) If you snack, plan the snack, and make it a nutritious snack.

You know you are full when:

(a) you feel full

(b) you feel nauseated

(c) there is pain in the back

(d) you are developing more GE reflux (heartburn)

Blockages or Obstruction of the Stoma

Because the opening from the upper stomach to the lower stomach is smaller than the pylorus, this stoma can easily become blocked with partially chewed food. All food should be chewed to a semi-solid liquid (the consistency of pudding) before swallowing it. Gulping down food will not work with this surgery. You cannot eat like Bert. Bert is my dog. Bert used to leave food in his dish, which my other dog, Ernie, would eat. Then we had Bert castrated—no more testicles but a great appetite (who says obesity isn't hormonal?). When you give Bert anything to eat, he takes three quick chews and swallows. If Bert were to have a VBG, he would have to learn to eat much more slowly.

If you do not chew your food properly a large piece of meat or vegetable can block the stoma. There are a several tricks for getting food unstuck. One way is to vomit it up. There are better ways, however, such as drinking a few sips of a highly-carbonated beverage. This will sometimes force the food through the stoma. (When food gets stuck in the esophagus, doctors sometimes prescribe "fizzies.") If some meat has stuck in there, you can try taking in some meat tenderizer (1/3 teaspoon of tenderizer in two teaspoons of water. Retry in a half an hour if necessary). If this does not work, a gastroenterologist will probably have to remove the blockage. If you go to the emergency room, please do not let them also give you contrast. The gastroenterologist will want to scope you first and if your gut is full of contrast, it will obscure the view. The gastroenterologist can remove those food bolus products and, if necessary, can enlarge the stoma.

If you develop an ulcer in the stoma, you may need to be on some medicine for the ulcer, such as Pepcid®, Prevacid®, or some such acid-blocking agent. Generally you will be on these medicines for at least six weeks, sometimes longer.

Eat a Balanced Diet, Just Less of It

The VBG is a simple tool that will allow you to eat a normal diet. There is nothing difficult here, just simple eating. While you need to have a diet high in protein after some surgeries, this surgery allows you to eat a diverse diet—but you will be able to eat less and be satisfied.

The pouch depends on solid food to distend it. If you are eating foods that are not solid, you are not using your new tool. Foods that we allow early post-op do not work later. For example, yogurt is a good food, but it will not keep you satisfied and full for long. Mashed potatoes have a lot of nutritional value, go down easily, but also go through the stoma easily. Again, there are no bad foods, just bad quantities of foods. This is the time to learn how to eat a balanced meal. Your pouch will enlarge, and that is a good thing. You will still be able enjoy eating more food, but the key to staying healthy and losing weight is in having a balanced diet.

Once again, the key to successful weight loss with the VBG surgery is to have a balanced diet with low-glycemic index carbohydrates and high-quality protein. Enjoy a balanced meal, feel full, and lose weight.

The VBG has stood the test of time. It works because it combines a simple restrictive component. It works best when patients are informed, learn what foods to eat and what foods will not work. VBG provides a sense of satiety and control over food that you couldn't enjoy before.

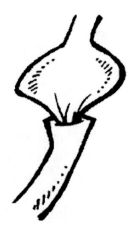

Six

Rules of the Pouch

Post-op Rules for the Patient with the Pouch

Roux-en-Y (RNY) Instructions

New RNY terms to learn during this time:

Pouch – This is the upper portion of the stomach. This is where your food goes. It will hold about one ounce, or 30 cc. If you have the micro-pouch, it will hold half that amount. If you had the BPD, then it can hold up to 8 ounces. Over time, this pouch will stretch, but how much it will stretch is up to you. If you eat too much, you can stretch this pouch to the size of your stomach—and then you will lose one of the components of this operation, the ability to eat less and be satisfied.

The lower stomach has been seperated from the upper stomach, or pouch, either by stapling or transection.

Anastomosis – This is the opening we surgeons create between the stomach and the small intestine. The other name for this is the "stoma." Technically, a stoma is the opening, and the anastomosis is the connection, but this may be more information than you need. This anastomosis is about half of an inch in diameter when we make it. In the first few weeks after surgery, it will swell and become smaller.

Satiety – Feeling full, no hunger. You feel full several minutes *after* you are actually full. If your pouch holds 30 cc (one ounce), you can put 30 cc of food in it, and you won't feel full for about five minutes. Try this one at home. Measure 30 cc, or one ounce of cottage cheese or tuna fish. Eat it and wait for a few minutes. That feeling you have—that is satiety, or *feeling full*. Of course, if you have a micro-pouch, then you will find that it takes half the amount to feel full.

Liquids do not produce this feeling. Why? Liquids will go through the pouch quickly, and into the small bowel. They don't cause the wall of the pouch to stretch, so you can drink a lot of liquids without a problem. However, you cannot, and should not gulp liquids.

Some bariatric surgeons refer to the new anatomy, the small pouch, as a tool that you can use to help learn new eating habits.

Measure Twice, Eat Once–Don't Vomit

Every time you sit down to eat, you must measure what you eat. The pouch has a limited amount of space so if you overfill it, you can either stretch the pouch or vomit.

RNY goals for the first few weeks:

(1) Learn to eat to the point of being satisfied without feeling full. Measure everything you eat.

(2) Start a moderate walking program to facilitate weight loss.

(3) Avoid food that causes diarrhea, vomiting, or discomfort.

(4) Learn to eat slowly and enjoy the food.

(5) Only eat foods that go through a straw until you reach the next phase.

(6) Time your meals, even if they are liquid. Enjoy them. Sit down for

them. The meal should take at least 5 minutes but no more than 30 minutes.

(7) Measure everything you put in your pouch. (You won't always do this, but for the first six weeks, you will). Learn how much you can hold, and don't exceed that amount. Eventually you will be able to measure your food with your eyes.

(8) Even though you haven't transitioned to regular food yet, make certain that you set aside at least three times a day when you act like you are eating a meal—even if it is one ounce of pureed haddock. This will help reinforce good habits so you don't get into a routine of grazing.

RNY foods to avoid:

- carbonated beverages (the carbonation may stretch your pouch)
- ice cream
- beverages containing sugar
- anything that cannot fit through a straw
- watch Nutra-Sweet carefully (in some patients it stimulates an appetite)

RNY liquids allowed:

See Appendix One.

RNY - A Look at Your New Anatomy

Your stomach is sore and tender from the surgery. The anastomosis has to heal; the only thing holding it together is staples and sutures. After surgery, everything swells, which means you have to be careful of how much you drink. Also, be careful not to eat anything solid. Can you screw it up? Yes, so you have to learn satiety. Drink only one-third of a medicine cup full at a time and no more. If you stuff yourself, bad things can happen. It takes six full weeks for the anastomosis to heal to 60-percent of its strength. So, if you drink too much you can disrupt the staple lines and cause a leak.

Vomiting

Vomiting will happen after surgery. The stomach is upset from the surgery, and even if you follow instructions to the letter, you might occasionally vomit. Some patients are lucky, however, and never have this problem. Some vomiting is normal but persistent vomiting is not normal or expected and your surgeon needs to hear from you if this is a problem.

RNY - Graduation from Clear Liquids to Full

This happens once you are able to tolerate the clear liquids and have demonstrated you can regulate them in the hospital under strict supervision. You should be able to drink one and one-half to 2 quarts (32-48 oz) a day of clear liquids. If for some reason you cannot, you may need to have nutrition through a vein. If your doctors put in a gastrostomy tube, you may have to be fed through this tube for a long period of time. Once you can tolerate clear liquids, you will start on a meal schedule starting with things like Boost®, Carnation Instant Breakfast®, or some equivalent mix.

Graduation from Full Liquids to Puree

Yippee! Real food

The theory is that liquids can wash food out of the pouch, allowing you to eat more. Now like all theories, we held this as absolute for years, and now we have discovered this isn't the case. But, if you gulp liquids down, to force down food, you can force it out of your pouch. It is also possibility is that the food won't wash out, and you will either vomit or stretch your pouch. A safe habit is to drink before you eat, and not to drink again until an hour after you eat. Now this might only apply the first few weeks after surgery. Later on, this rule can be relaxed. Early on, the pouch is swollen from surgery and it is difficult to tell when you are satisfied and when you are not.

Terms to Learn During This Period

High-quality protein: This is protein that is low in fat. High-quality proteins are easy to digest, provide the building blocks that you need to heal from your surgery, and don't have fats that are associated with cardiac disease. Typical examples of high-quality proteins include tofu, egg whites, whey proteins, fish, and shellfish. Most patients find they enjoy tuna fish (either in the foil packet or water-packed) or shrimp as a good source of protein during this time. These high-quality proteins are not only healthy, but they digest much easier than proteins such as red meat, fatty meats, poultry, or other proteins. In contrast to high-quality proteins, which not only contain little fat but also have essential amino acids, there are low-quality proteins. The most common are those found in gelatin. While gelatin is essentially fat-free, the proteins in it are not useful for rebuilding your body after surgery.

Protein powders: Okay, I admit it. I can be a bit of a skeptic. I always tell patients to receive protein from food instead of a shake or a drink, but enough of my patients have used them and benefited from them, that now I am a believer. (Isn't there a Monkees song about that?) If you go into most nutritional stores or the health section of the grocery store, you will find an abundant source of protein powders and shakes. Whey protein is easier to digest than soy protein. Egg white is a great source of protein. Some protein drinks can cause some discomfort such as gas and loose stools. I recommend Isopure® and several others.

For the amount of protein you should have, see Appendix One.

Good Protein Choices

Low-fat cottage cheese (it comes in handy containers that are easy to carry to lunch), custard, and low-fat yogurt are good protein choices. A number of puddings are made especially for patients (Resource®, Sustacal®), or liquid scrambled eggs or Eggbeaters® (that you can pour out into nice portions). Some people like to use baby food during this time (comes in neat containers, but you do receive some interesting looks as you spoon it out). The important thing is that you have only puree and soft foods, something that will go easy on the pouch and not lead to vomiting.

Soft Foods to Real Food

For weeks now since your surgery, you have been giving your stomach a rest by carefully avoiding certain foods. Your stomach is still a bit tender, probably not ready to have a steak, but you are pretty tired of protein shakes. Now is the time to test your stomach a bit. This is a transition phase from soft foods to regular foods. This isn't the time to go from yogurt to steak with vegetables, but it is time to test things a little. Some soft foods go down well, and some don't. Moist chicken works well. Chicken or turkey breast, which is a bit drier, might not be as good. Chicken salad works great, and can be a good source of protein. Put the blender away, and start to experiment just a bit with your diet.

You will also decrease the number of meals you have from five to seven a day to only three or four. Every surgeon has his or her own way of getting you through this phase and their own time schedule, but typically this transition occurs around the sixth week.

Schedule

Clear liquid	Full liquid	Puree	Soft	Regular
In hospital	1st week	4 weeks	2 weeks	After 6 weeks

Goals for Six Weeks to Six Months

(1) Remember the size of your pouch and don't overfill it. Solids fill you up, stick in the stomach, and slowly trickle out. Remember, the feeling of "satiety" isn't instantaneous. As you transition to solid foods, it is better to have a bit less than you think will fill the pouch than to over-fill it. If you want the pouch to stretch, overfill it. If you want to vomit, overfill it.

(2) If you cannot tolerate a food today, don't worry. The typical progression of foods that the stomach will tolerate goes from fish, to foul, to beef (swim, fly, walk). If you cannot tolerate something today, try it later.

(3) Cut your food to the size of half a pea and chew it thoroughly. The stoma is a bit less than half an inch, and if something gets stuck in there, then you will either vomit it out, or your gastroenterologist will have to take it out with an endoscope. If you don't learn to cut up your food and then to chew your food, you will be quite uncomfortable.

(4) Three or four meals a day is the rule. A meal should last no less than five minutes or no more than 30 minutes. Sit down and enjoy the meal. You will be eating a lot less than everyone else in the family, so take your time and enjoy the company.

(5) Do not skip meals to accelerate weight loss. So you are not a breakfast eater and never have been. Learn to eat it. Plan what you will eat, eat high-quality protein, and enjoy your food. Snacks happen because of hunger and hunger happens when you have missed a meal. Think—did missing breakfast really help you lose weight in the past? What you eat in the morning makes you feel full for the afternoon.

(6) Get a smaller plate, a smaller fork, a smaller spoon. You will eat less, you will have smaller portions, and you have to cut it smaller. Using utensils designed for this purpose makes sense. Small portions are a key to weight loss, and now it is enforced.

(7) There is a growing body of evidence that sips of water with your meal will not wash out the food. This may be a myth that is slowly leaving the weight loss surgery literature. In a survey of 30 patients who reached their goal weight with RNY, and maintained that for at least

two years, all of them sipped some liquids with meals. However, none of them "gulped" their liquids. None of them drank and ate at the same time during the first 12 weeks. The pouch requires different treatment during that time.

(8) Drink a lot between meals. Most RNY patients complain of constipation, and most constipation comes from not drinking enough. Now, I have never had a patient tell me that I was right. My patients all say that they drink plenty. When they measure what they drink, they find they don't drink as much as they should. Drinking water or sugar-free liquids also decreases appetite.

First it sustains you, now we want you to avoid it

For the first six weeks you lived on pureed foods, soups, and liquid drinks. Now that you are eating solids, soups and pureed foods become something to avoid. You may need to go back to soups and pureed foods for a period of time if you cannot tolerate solids, but that is a separate issue. Solids empty differently than liquids.

Solids provide a sense of fullness that you may have been missing in the first couple of weeks. So, as your stomach can tolerate these solid foods, you will notice a new sense of satiety with smaller portions. Your stomach will grind away at the solids and eventually they will empty into the intestines. Liquids, soups, and many puree foods go passively through the stomach. Strange to think of it this way but it is kind of a weaning process. You have your teeth back, your stomach is getting ready for solid foods, and it is time to graduate from one and put the other behind you.

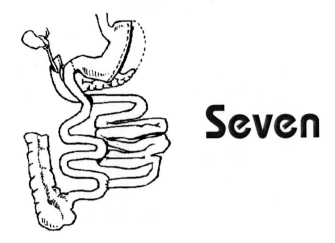

Seven

Rules for DS Patients

Post-Op Duodenal Switch Tips

Post-op duodenal switch patients have a bit larger stomach, and one that functions better than most other weight loss surgery patients. Their diet progression is usually more rapid than other patients; however, the stomach is still a bit tender at first. Here is the typical progression:

Clear liquid	Full liquid	Puree	Soft	Regular
The day after surgery if the upper GI is clear	If clear liquids are tolerated then this is attempted. However lactose should be avoided for several months	Often for the first two weeks after surgery, although some progress through this in the hospital	In hospital, transition to regular diet	Some progress to a regular diet while in the hospital, others will progress more slowly, depending on the doctor

Do Not Top Off

Everyone is surprised at how small their stomach is after surgery. Often it is difficult to imagine that, with this four-ounce stomach, only a couple of fork loads of food will fill you up. Do not exceed what will fill you. If you do, you will find a terrible discomfort level, and that can be manifested in a number of ways: you may feel pain in the back or the shoulders, you may feel nauseated, or you may feel as if something is stuck in your throat.

With DS you will have a larger "pouch" or stomach than with the one-ounce RNY, lap-band, or VBG, but four ounces is not that much larger. If you eat or drink a bit more than you think you should, nothing good will come of it. You may be uncomfortable, start to vomit, or rupture your staple line. So, just like at the gas station—don't top it off (those of you from Oregon and New Jersey will not understand this as you do not have self-serve gasoline pumps, so while we acknowledge your superiority, please humor us here). Just because we say you have a four-ounce stomach does not mean you can eat four ounces—when you had a 50-ounce stomach, did you eat a 50-ounce steak?

Getting in the Protein

The stomach can be quite picky the first few weeks after surgery. Do not force protein at the risk of vomiting. There are a lot of sources of protein that you can use. Sometimes, and I hate to admit this, the only way you can get in enough protein early on is through drinks or supplements.

Jim was a wonderful patient of mine whose wife kind of ruled the roost—in fact, there was no question about it. When he was getting ready to go home from the hospital, he just didn't feel like having the typical hospital lunch (which was turkey breast that had been dried out and cooked until it was unidentifiable by most pathologists). His wife insisted that he eat it, otherwise horrible things would happen to him (after all, she took seriously that protein was important). He didn't eat the turkey and I assured her that if the stomach doesn't feel like eating, it is probably better to give it a rest than to eat something and vomit later.

Food Intolerance

Can't we all just get along?

You will find patients who can, and will, eat anything. If they have an iron deficiency they will eat rusty nails, if they need more protein, they will chew the hide off a cow. But most patients, after surgery, find they are a bit touchy about some foods. What goes down easily one day may not go down the next. As you re-introduce foods into your diet, go slow. Don't try the new recipe that combines a lot of new foods at once (the Ostrich-alligator casserole may be a bit much at first). Try one new thing at a time. If the duck doesn't sit well—wait a week before you have quackers with your crackers again.

Lactose Intolerance

Lactose intolerance is very common after duodenal switch surgery. Milk and milk products should be reintroduced in a gradual manner. Generally, the more firm the consistency of the dairy product, the easier it is to tolerate—hard cheese is tolerated where whole milk may cause cramping and diarrhea. There are tablets that help you digest lactose, but it is sometimes best to avoid milk for a few months. Then, as with all foods, go slowly.

Swim, Fly, and Then Walk

Ketchikan salmon are the best fish to eat

As with all weight loss surgeries, the progression of food is swim, fly, and then walk. If it is in the water and swims, you can probably tolerate it pretty well after surgery. The second month you can expand to food that flies, and finally, as you start walking more—go out and catch a bison. Now there are some unique exceptions to this, and the first has to do with seafood. Do not fry your seafood. Fried and battered seafood will not sit well after surgery.

The next exception comes from someone who was born in the salmon capitol of the world—get fresh fish. One day I was visiting my best friend in Los Angeles. He took me out to "the finest" seafood place in the city, so I asked about the salmon. I was assured that this was fresh, caught that day, but when the plate came and I smelled it, I sent it back and ordered the steak.

Since we are talking about salmon: do not EVER eat farm-raised salmon. I know this is an editorial, but it is *my* book, and I don't like farm-raised salmon. Salmon that is wild and caught fresh is the best salmon you can buy. Farm-raised salmon is not a substitute (sometimes this is called "Atlantic raised" salmon). One more story. Once while I was having dinner with some friends in San Francisco at one of my favorite Italian restaurants, the waiter told us that salmon was the fresh fish catch-of-the-day. Three of us were from Alaska and we immediately asked if it was caught or raised, the waiter assured us it was not raised, but caught, so the three of us ordered it as an appetizer. It was raised, not caught. You can not fool an Alaskan about salmon.

Raised salmon and wild salmon are not the same. They don't taste the same, and raised salmon is artificially colored. So, if you hate salmon, try some salmon that is freshly caught, like troll-caught out of Ketchikan, from the Kenai River, the Russian River, or the Copper River (which means it was trying to get to my brother's house along the river). Salmon is a great fish. If it is fresh and caught in the wild, it will be a wonderful dish. If it is farm raised, save your money and buy some tuna fish instead. Besides, I have a lot of friends in Alaska who are commercial fishermen, which is a very difficult way to make a living. The "farm-raised" salmon has almost shut down their industry, as restaurants have purchased the less-expensive salmon. So, if you go out to a restaurant, and the salmon was not "caught," order the steak.

Beans are a great source of protein and have a low-glycemic index; however, they can be a source of gas. Beano® is a great product, and will decrease the malodor. So beans are not a food intolerance—just a social one.

The first month proteins that are tolerated well include:

- seafood – fish and shrimp are easy on the stomach
- tuna fish (it is a seafood, but sometimes we don't think of it that way)
- tofu (there are some great tofu recipes. This is a high quality protein)
- Bocca® burgers – available at most supermarkets and are a ready source of protein

- cottage cheese – a great source of protein. It is soft and easily fills you. Some new products have fruit in them for flavor. Low-fat cottage cheese is preferred.
- egg whites – a great source of protein (you don't need the yolks) and you can use them in a variety of ways.

If the stomach is just too tender and you are vomiting, talk to your surgeon. Vomiting is not the desired result (this is not the super-model diet—eat, vomit, eat, vomit). Some patients find that they must have a little food on their stomach to soak up the acid, such as a cracker or a chewable antacid. Do not overstuff your stomach. You may only be able tolerate a forkful or two before you have to stop. Sometimes during the first month, you may have to take protein drinks to get in the protein you need. Over time your stomach will stretch, so don't be alarmed if you cannot eat as much as you think you should, but do not attempt to overfill it.

The second month - proteins can expand to poultry items
- chicken (some can tolerate this the first month)
- duck (always a favorite)
- deli-meats

Third month - ready for red meats
- beef – ground, slow-cooked, tenderized. Fried foods can be difficult to tolerate, as can meats that are dry-cooked too long.
- elk –a great source of protein

Sometimes the Food Doesn't Taste Right

Sometimes after surgery, it is difficult to get in the protein simply because you have lost a taste for it. Your tongue wants something with more "spice" or something tart (not a Pop Tart, and not an English version of a tart). Spice is not hard on the stomach. Contrary to the old belief that spices might contribute to ulcers, they don't. So add balsamic vinegar, capers, salsa (which is right up our alley here in the Southwest), pickles, or olives—these all add a bit of flavor to the food, make it easier to go down, and wake up the taste buds. The other is sushi—forget the rice, but add some of the ginger. Not only will your taste buds wake up, but also your sinuses will clear up faster than you can imagine. Peppers—hot, moderate, or mild, can also help spice up protein.

Beware of the Carbohydrate Trap

Carbohydrates go down very easily—mashed potatoes, chips, ice cream. Some patients fool themselves into thinking that it is better to have these foods than it is to have nothing. This is the carbohydrate trap. Until your BMI reaches 25, potatoes are a good thing to look forward to occasionally but they are not a substitute for protein. Soft foods do go down easily, but there are better choices: tuna fish with mayonnaise, chicken salad, cottage cheese, and broiled Cornish game hens. There are two reasons to avoid high-glycemic index carbohydrates in the early post-operative period:

(1) You need the protein. You need protein to heal your wounds. Surgery requires that we cut things and sew them back together. Protein is required as a building block for healing. The less protein you eat the more likely you are to develop a hernia or other post-operative problems.

(2) Carbohydrates inhibit weight loss. You have a limited amount of room in your stomach. Using that for carbohydrates will slow your weight loss. Some carbohydrates are better for you than others—see Appendix One for this list.

Fruits, fruit juices, and sodas contain a lot of carbohydrates, and these inhibit weight loss. So, be cautious of these. Anything that isn't a protein should be used in moderation.

Don't Eat Yourself

—or, self-cannibalization

Any time you don't take in enough protein, your muscle tissue and "lean body mass" will start to break down. You will feel weak, lethargic, be lightheaded, and have nausea. The most common time this occurs is right after surgery, which is also the most dangerous. Protein is needed to heal the anastomosis, to heal the incision, and for the increased energy requirements your body has after surgery. Swelling of the ankles and calves is another sign of protein malnutrition. It is normal immediately after surgery to have swelling, but this should resolve a few days after you return home.

There are special machines to measure lean body mass, and body fat percentage, and these are helpful to determine if your weight loss is coming from fat or from muscle tissue. We use the Tanita (http://www.tanita.com) body fat scale in our office to monitor patients after surgery.

Grazing Is Okay for Cows

—but not for patients

If you are taking longer than 30 minutes to eat a meal, you are grazing. Grazing will kill any weight loss surgery, including the duodenal switch. While we want you to get protein into your body, we don't want you to graze. So, eat three meals a day and make certain that they are high-protein meals. It is easy to have a bit, wait, and have a bit more, wait—but that is gazing. Ever wonder how we would do the duodenal switch on an animal with five stomachs?

Fats May Not Be Absorbed

—but they are still not your friends

With the duodenal switch, a lot less fat is absorbed. That is the good news. The bad news is that the fat comes out like an oil slick in Prince William Sound. The first few months, avoiding high fat foods will make you less prone to loose stools, gas, diarrhea, and accidents. While fats make food taste good—they give a creamy texture to fine ice creams, avoiding fats the first few months will help you avoid some embarrassing moments. Some patients even report "oil slicks" on their undergarments so, put the bacon away, trim the fat off the meat, and concentrate on those proteins that are "high quality," or low in fat and high in protein, such as shrimp, fish, tofu and other soy products.

How to Prepare Foods

Chef Terry will be available on the food channel soon enough, but until then, or until we come to our chapters about menus and diets, here are a few simple tips to make your food easy to tolerate:

- Do not deep-fry the foods. Fried foods do not go down well, and the fats can cause some problems. For whatever reason, the stomach doesn't like fried foods the first few months.

- Do not overcook the food. I had a neighbor who thought the only way to cook a steak was to make sure it was overcooked. His steaks were useful to repair side panels on automobiles. Dried-out, well-done meat does not sit well on your stomach after this surgery, nor do other well-done foods.

- Keep the food moist: a slow cooker (known to most of us as a Crock Pot®) is the gift that keeps on giving. You get a slow cooker for your wedding, it stays in the original box, and when the next couple gets married, you pass it on to them, kind of like fruitcake. Keeping meat on the moist side is best, and using the slow cooker is a wonderful way to do that.

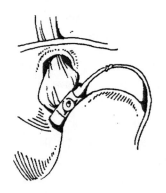

Eight

Post-Op Bandsters

The Band, and What to Expect Following Surgery

The adjustable laparoscopic band (ALB) is usually placed in the abdomen with very little or no fluid in the band. The foreign models (mid-band, Swedish band, and others) might have some fluid placed in them, but mainly we are discussing the lap-band from Inamed®. Your surgeon wants the band to heal in place, allowing your body to get used to this new foreign object before you begin putting food into your stomach. Typically, this means the diet progression in the ALB is different from, and much slower than, diets of other weight loss surgery patients.

Vomiting is the enemy here, as early repeated vomiting can cause displacement of the band. If your band becomes displaced, you will need to go back to the operating room to have it adjusted. So, follow your doctor's instructions closely about diet progression.

The day after surgery, or later in the afternoon on the day of surgery, you will get a barium swallow (this is where you go to the x-ray room and drink some chalk-tasting fluid). This swallow will show the surgeon that fluid is going through the banded area, and that the band is in its proper position.

Some patients will feel as if they cannot even swallow their saliva. They will stay in the hospital a few days for IV fluids while the swelling goes down. This can occur even though barium goes through the banded area into the lower stomach. Medications can be given to dry out the secretions and to make the stomach work a little better, but this is a temporary condition that will clear up on its own if given a little time.

Week 1-2	Week 2-3	Band fill	Week 3 and on
See the clear liquid diet recommendations. Sip from 1-ounce cups, and sip no more than 1/3 of that cup at a time.	Full liquid diet. Avoid swelling foods: no bread, no rice, and no pasta. Avoid fiber.	Go back to clear liquids for 2 days— sip, sip, and sip. Do not tempt your band at this time.	Go to a puree diet, and advance to soft then to solid foods. But, the foods must be small bites.

Progression of the diet for patients who have the lap-band surgery varies greatly. Some doctors allow you to have a full liquid diet by the second week and to slowly increase your intake from that point. Again, the enemy here is vomiting, and early introduction of too much food can cause severe vomiting.

The first few weeks after ALB surgery, unlike other weight loss surgeries, are not meant for weight loss. This is an adjustment period for you to learn to use your tool. Learn to take small sips of clear liquids. Give your stomach a chance to get used to the band. This is not the time to experiment with food or to try something new. This is the time to sit back and enjoy a liquid diet while allowing the band to scar into its new home. After the second week, you can begin the full liquids. Foods like yogurt go down quite well. Some surgeons consider yogurt a "clear liquid" and will allow it the first week.

Filling the Band

The stoma is closing, all aboard...

Most surgeons place the lap-band into the abdomen without fluid in the balloon (a fill) and wait several weeks (sometimes six to eight) before the first fill. More often than not, you will feel a restriction even though no fluid has been placed in the band. It is also normal *not* to feel a restriction of the stomach at first. By restricted, we mean that you will feel full with less, usually less than a cup of food will fill you. Without the restriction, your stomach can accommodate a small water buffalo. The initial restriction you feel is just swelling from the surgery. This swelling reaches its maximum at about one week after the surgery and can last for up to six or seven weeks. As the swelling begins to decrease and the band has healed into place, your surgeon may put some saline into the port, causing the balloon to fill, which will restrict your outflow stoma.

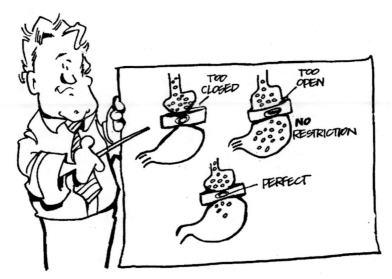

The lap-band fits around the top part of the stomach and is adjustable. If we tighten it too much no food will get through. If we do not "fill" it, then there will be no restriction and you will not feel full with less food. The trick is to have a "fill" that tightens it "just right." That way, you feel a restriction with a bit of food and the food is allowed to go slowly into the lower stomach, keeping you full longer.

The first fill may not be very much (just a few cc's of saline), but it may have a profound effect on how you feel. Filling the balloon will tighten the stoma, so you will feel quite restricted where you didn't before. A bite or two will fill you up and you will have no appetite for more. Some surgeons do the first fill in x-ray while you drink some dye (barium). This way, they can close the band, watch the barium sit in your esophagus, and then gently open it so there is the correct amount of restriction. Other surgeons will do the fill in their office and judge the fill according to the patient's response.

Before the fill, it is best not to have anything but water on your stomach. Every surgeon has a different protocol for this. Most will ask that you have nothing to eat after midnight but will allow you to drink water up to two hours before your fill.

The goal is to design your pouch and stoma so that you are satisfied with a small amount of food. There is an art to filling the band. The first time it is filled, you will feel a restriction to the intake, then as time goes on it goes away. That is the time for another fill. A lot of this will depend on the protocol that your surgeon uses. If he does the first fill in x-ray, you will feel a restriction. If he "fills" in the office, he may want to creep up on the restriction.

Every surgeon has a different protocol for filling the band. In Tijuana, my friends like to do their fill in x-ray, but the cost of the x-ray and the fill is only $150. Again, the cost savings of medical care in Mexico is passed on to the patient. In the United States, x-ray can be an expensive option, so many surgeons will adjust the band in the office.

Remember—after your adjustment, the rule is "clear liquid diet" for two days. There will be some swelling and your body needs to get used to your new anatomy. Vomiting can still displace the band. If that happens, it means you will have to go back to the operating room to have the band put back in place.

Foods to Avoid Early-On

—the swellers (like Mama's leg on a hot Georgia day)

Some foods may swell in your pouch and cause problems. These are bread, rice, pasta, and some cereals. These must be avoided early on in order to allow the stomach to heal. Fresh hot bread sounds delicious, but it can swell in your pouch and make you very uncomfortable. Broccoli and asparagus tips can give you fits so it is best to avoid them (remember the first President Bush? You can be like him and refuse to eat broccoli—okay, maybe not, but avoid the broccoli anyway). Some patients, if they chew the vegetables well, have no problem with any of these items. Proceed with caution. Again, the enemy is vomiting. If you vomit or feel uncomfortable with a certain food, then avoid that food for a while. Really, there are a lot of food choices in the world, so don't feel deprived. Just wait.

This is a Solid Diet

—so, no mushy foods allowed

Having the band means you can have a solid diet and be satisfied with a few ounces of food. You should not have "mushy" foods. Foods like yogurt, mashed potatoes, and other soft foods will not fill your upper pouch or keep you satisfied. They will go through your pouch, and you will feel hungry again.

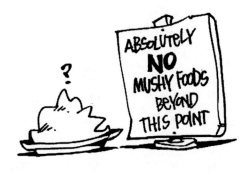

Early on, those foods may feel good to your pouch. As with most surgeries, there will be times when your stomach just doesn't feel like having certain foods. That is okay. The key to the success of this surgery is that it allows you to eat mostly solid foods and regular meals. With that small amount of food you are satisfied.

Patients with the adjustable band do not have the same diet requirements as those who have had other types of weight loss surgery and they can have a more "normal" diet. We encourage patients to consult with a nutritionist before surgery to learn what and how to eat. You can have a bit of everything on the menu, but in smaller amounts. Do not skip meals. Have three meals a day about five hours apart.

Drinking and Eating

Typically, if you have a good restriction, one cup of food will fill you and you will be quite satisfied. Again, this is dependent on having a good fill. If you are able to eat more than one cup full and still feel hungry, you might need a fill. The band is similar to the VBG and the RNY gastric bypass in that liquid may force foods from the upper pouch into the lower stomach, resulting in hunger. Traditionally surgeons have advocated "don't drink" for at least an hour after eating. This is not always the case. Most patients find they cannot eat without drinking a bit of liquid with it. Sipping small amounts of liquid with some foods will not force food into the lower stomach. So, if you sip when you eat, that is fine, but DO NOT GULP. The secret to feeling full is to change your eating habits—chew your food well, swallow, and sip water or other liquids.

Important tips:

- Cut food into a piece the size of your little fingernail
- Chew each bite at least ten times
- If you need some liquid—sip, do not gulp
- Limit your liquid with a meal to one cup at a time

You need to be aware of your water intake. Remember, two quarts a day is all you need. Early on, when the stomach is tender, you will need to sip water all the time. Some patients find they can drink warm or hot liquids, while others find they can only tolerate very cold liquids. This is an individual preference, and you will need to experiment with it. Water can also be a good tool to make you feel satisfied. Between meals, drinking a lot of water will keep you feeling full and prevent constipation. But don't forget—after the band is placed you must always sip, don't gulp.

Some surgeons do not want their patients to eat and drink at the same time—ever. If that is the case, then you should start drinking liquids no sooner than 60 minutes after eating a meal. Start by sipping. If you feel full, wait a bit until you can sip some liquids. Meals should be no more than five hours apart, so after three hours (and this is a reason to set the clock) start drinking a lot of water or other liquids. Half-an-hour to fifteen minutes before your next meal, drink one to two cups of water (don't gulp). This is called water loading, it will make you feel less like you have to eat and drink at the same time and it will allow you to feel much fuller after eating just a cup of food. Water is also a calorie-free way to feel full if you get quite hungry between meals. Instead of reaching for that donut, have some water. You probably need the water anyway (we do here in the Sonoron Desert).

Commandment Number One

—Know the size of thy pouch and do not overfill it

Your eyes may be bigger than your stomach—literally. As you advance to solid food, measure what you eat and learn the meaning of "satiety." Some of you will feel the restriction right away, while others will not feel any restriction. If you have a good fill, you will discover what it takes to feel full. If you are being adjusted slowly, then you need to measure your food first. So measure your food twice, and eat once—you do not want to stretch your pouch, and you do not want to vomit. The last thing you want is to go back to surgery because the band slipped.

Changing Behaviors—Oiy

Once you feel the restriction you will have a great feeling of control over food. People are often frustrated and depressed at their inability to stop eating before they get a good restriction. Be patient. The beauty of the band is that we can adjust it, and often we can do this in the doctor's office. You discover it doesn't take much to fill you up before you put the plate away. For many, this is a new feeling and one that gives you the control over food you never had before. Your biology is now working for you instead of against you.

You should use smaller utensils to eat, cut your food well before you put it in your mouth, and chew well. Shoveling food in and following it with a water chaser will not work with this band, and if you try that, you will be quite unhappy. You will be uncomfortable, sick, nauseated and may vomit. Old habits are hard to break and new habits are hard to learn, but this is one you have to learn. Your food must be cut to the size of your little fingernail before you put it into your mouth. Then you have to chew at least ten times—however, you do not need to practice Fletcherization.

Variety is the spice of life and of foods. My father eats the salad first, then the meat, then the vegetable or fruit, and finally dessert. He is very regimented—and at age 78 looks great (Mom thinks so, but after 52 years of looking at the guy it is nice to know she finds him interesting). That isn't the point. The point is that you will not be eating a lot of anything, so have a bit of variety with every small forkful. Many will advocate eating the meat first and then the vegetables.

Speaking of forks—if you are using anything larger than a salad fork, you may feel as if you are not eating enough food. Using small utensils has two benefits: the first is that you cannot shove a lot of food in with a smaller fork or spoon. The second is psychological: your subconscious is programmed to see a spoonful or a forkful as a unit. Now you can have a larger fork and eat more food in fewer bites, or a smaller fork and eat less food in more bites and feel full with less. So—break out the small stuff. If some snooty person tells you that you are using the wrong fork, tell them to "Fork off!"

Pregnancy – Getting in the Nutrition

Eat for Two, Not Four

The beauty of the band is that if you become pregnant, the band can be emptied to allow you to take in more calories. While we prefer that patients wait two years after the band is placed before becoming pregnant, oftentimes that does not happen. Sometimes, once the restrictive nature of the band is lifted, you eat a lot more than you should, so even though you don't have the band filled, watch your portions. I am not an obstetrical doctor, but it makes sense that you do not need to gain 90 pounds with your pregnancy—honest.

A – Stands for Adjust, Not Absent

The advantage of the adjustable laparoscopic band is that it can be adjusted. This means you need to keep in touch with your surgeon. For those who have had the band placed in other countries, you might have to go back for fills. A friend of mine, Dr. Ariel Ortiz Lagardere, has an extensive network of friends in the United States who are more than happy to see his patients and offer adjustments. Don't you love Latin names? I mean, how wide are the columns in their phonebooks? If you have your band done in a foreign country you must make sure someone in the United States will take care of it, and that can be a problem. Surgeons who have good reputations and are well-trained, like my long-named friend, have no problem having us fill them. But be prepared—the first fill we do for another surgeon is done in the x-ray suite and costs more than ones done in the office. This shows us if the band is in place and allows us to do a fill with precision. If you have a band that is not approved for use in the United States, it is unlikely that you will find any surgeon willing to fill that device. That is an unfortunate reality in our litigious society.

Filling the band is a fairly simple process, but it does involve using special equipment and needles. Knowing when to fill is the trick, not how to fill, and this is where you need to have a good relationship with your surgeon. Sometimes you lose some weight and then the band becomes a bit loose. This is the advantage of the band. You can have a quick fill and regain that feeling of satiety with a small meal. When the band is placed around the stomach, it incorporates a bit of fat. As this fat disappears (along with other fat in your body) the band becomes a bit loose, and it is time for another fill. It might not take much to fill, just a bit. Typically, after the first year or two, fills may not be needed. Some patients periodically require a bit of a fill for several years. Keep in touch with your surgeon. It is important, as they can offer an adjustment and get you back on the road to weight loss.

Do Not Top Off

–applies to gas tanks and laparoscopic bands

Putting too much fluid in the band can cause discomfort to you. Too much pressure on the stomach can cause a perforation, so most surgeons will be a bit conservative. There is no pain with a band, but if there is pain after a fill, you need to call your surgeon immediately. While the adjustment will make you feel tight, and cause some heartburn, if you should wake up the next morning with pain, CALL. Your surgeon will probably need to remove some fluid from the band.

Oops–It's Stuck

Sometimes you cannot help it—you know better, but now something is stuck. You have vomited but it is not coming up. There are a couple of simple choices, but oftentimes this means your surgeon will have to empty the band to allow the food bolus to pass. Sometimes a bit of a carbonated beverage will allow the food bolus to pass but try this only under your surgeon's direction. As a rule, carbonation is not something we like to advocate but there are some exceptions. (Again, some surgeons think carbonation will stretch the pouch, and some don't think this will be a problem at all.) Do not do this without your surgeon's permission or intervention. As we said in an earlier chapter, radiologists use "fizzy" pills to remove a food bolus. If you have something stuck—make certain your surgeon is involved in the removal of it.

Preventing foods from getting stuck is a key to successful recovery from this surgery. You will be more comfortable following some simple rules than being uncomfortable and worrying whether the band has slipped.

PB – Know the Lingo...

A PB is a productive burp – there is also a BB – bandster burp. This is the lingo you will hear from patients everywhere who have had the band. If you have overeaten or didn't chew something well, or had something that just got stuck, you will have these burps. A PB is not quite vomiting, but still something that should be avoided—especially at the dinner table with others present. It can be quite embarrassing in company.

What Is Feeling Full?

This might be a new sensation for you. Once you have a good fill and feel "the restriction," you need to learn that sensation of fullness (satiety). This is a sensation to learn so you will not overfill. You don't want to have PB, you don't want to vomit, you don't want to feel uncomfortable. The best way to learn this is to experiment with some solid food like tuna. Have a tablespoon of food, and wait a few minutes. See if you can have another tablespoon and wait again. It takes your brain a few minutes to register that your stomach is stretched. Feel that, memorize that sensation and promise yourself to not overdo that again.

There Are No Bad Foods

–only bad quantities of food

There are no bad foods; there are only bad quantities of food. There are always those who will disagree with me, and sometimes talking to patients who have been successful at losing weight is like talking to alcoholics about an occasional glass of wine. I have some patients who have become religious in their avoidance of certain foods because they feel they are poison. Food really isn't poison unless you take too much of it (or it is spoiled). Remember the saying, "moderation in all things, including moderation." As with alcohol, some people can never just have a glass of wine, and some people cannot just have a bit of cake. You have to judge this for yourself. Obesity is a life-long disease for which surgery is only a tool.

The lap-band surgery provides a tool that can change as your body changes. This means after surgery you will eat a "normal diet." Now, it might take some education in order to learn what is normal but you certainly will be satisfied with less. The key to this surgery is in learning the meaning of "normal." Normal is not fast food, normal is not milkshakes. Normal is high-quality proteins (low-fat, or fats made from olive oil or fish) and low-glycemic index carbohydrates. You will not only eat healthy foods, you will achieve weight loss without feeling hungry, and that 3 o'clock candy bar won't tempt you.

Patients who have had either the small bowel or the duodenum bypassed, need to concentrate on protein first and take in up to 100 grams of protein a day. With the lap-band, there is no need to take in more than the recommended daily allowance (RDA). See Appendix One for details.

What to eat:

- normal foods
- high quality proteins (egg whites, fish, low fat cottage cheese, soy products)
- low-glycemic index carbohydrates
- vegetables
- fruits

The lap-band is the new revolution in the fight against obesity. It is a great tool, so use it well.

Proper aftercare cannot happen in the absence of self-advocacy.

—Melanie Magruder,

patient of Dr. Robert Rabkin

Part 4

Recipes & Meal Plans

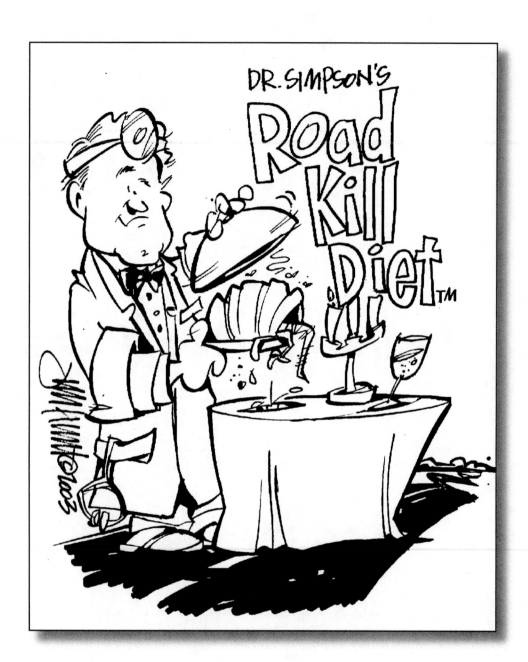

"Roadkill Diet"

Excerpts from "Roadkill Diet"

The following is an excerpt from my next book—*The Roadkill Diet: Post-Operative Weight Loss Surgery Patient's Guide.* This book is meant to be a guidebook for those patients who have had weight loss surgery and need some simple tips, menu plans, and recipes to get them out of a plateau and into weight loss. Now, while I love the title of the book—as does my illustrator, I am told that this isn't appropriate as a title so before publication we might be talked into changing the title of the book. Until then....

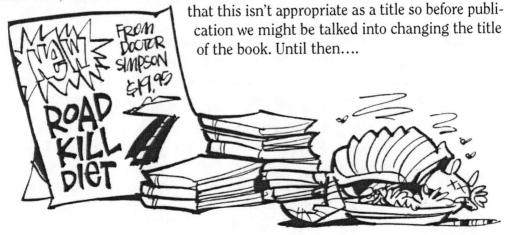

To Diet Or Not To Diet

Now that you are beyond the pain of the surgery, (or even if you are many years out from weight loss surgery), and want to lose more weight, you might ask, "Should I go back on Atkins or go to Weight-Watchers?" The answer is no and the reason is simple. Those diets are meant for people with a large stomach and a large appetite. Those diets are not designed for you. That is why we wrote this book—this book is a collection of menu plans and recipes from patients who have had success with weight loss surgery, a few celebrity chefs who altered favorite items for weight loss patients, and some of my favorite items. You have a tool—a smaller stomach or pouch, which has some specific needs. It might be stretched a bit, but you have a tool for weight loss. Now our goal is to get off that plateau and figure out what works best.

There are so many popular diets out there, but they all have one thing in common: they are boring. Hey, you made the ultimate sacrifice, you had some surgeon (like me) open you up and rearrange your guts so you could lose weight, and now you want to go back to one of these diets? You still have an advantage. You still have a small stomach, so let's have some variety, some flavor, some salsa! But before we jump into menus and recipes, let us review some old favorite diet plans and how they work.

The One-Food or One-Food Group Diet

The most famous diet, at least today, is the Atkins diet. It has been almost universally tried by all of my patients and misunderstood, perhaps even by the Atkins folks themselves. Robert Atkins made a great deal out of the body going into "ketosis" where it burns fat instead of turning food into fat. He had a complicated set of theories. None was ever proven, however. The reason you lose weight on that, or any low-carbohydrate diet, is simple—you don't eat as much.

Most diets have one thing in common: people eat less on them. If you eat less food, then you consume fewer calories, and if you consume fewer calories you will, in most circumstances, lose weight. With the Atkins diet, people don't lose weight because they are in ketosis, they lose weight because they consume less food than they did before going on this diet. This has been confirmed by a number of studies.

I Gained Weight On Atkins

–or, biology does not overcome the laws of physics

How is this possible? Heresy, I say. How can you gain weight on a diet that promises that you will lose weight if you avoid carbohydrates and eat meat? The great thing about writing this book for weight loss surgery patients is that most of them have been on this diet, or a variation of this diet, and they know, given their pre-operative anatomy, that they really did gain weight on a diet by following the diet. After all, when you have a stomach that can hold a small mammal, you know you can eat your way into ketotic weight-gain on the Atkins diet. Simply put, a calorie is a calorie is a calorie. It doesn't matter if you get the calorie from meat, from figs, from bread, or from alcohol. If you get a bunch of calories together, you will store them and if you store them, you will store them as fat. Yup, eat enough steak and you will gain weight.

If you are given only a single food, even if it is a food that you like, there is only so much of it that you can eat before you don't want anymore. I love steak—put a 16-ounce steak in front of me and I will consume 10 ounces of it and bring the rest home for Bert and Ernie. After 10 ounces, I am done with the steak, I can't eat anymore. So, if I am on a low-carbohydrate diet, you can bet that I am done with dinner. But, if I am not on that diet and you put a bunch of French fries with the steak, not only will I have my 10 ounces of steak, but I will also have four ounces of fries and maybe even think about dessert. Let us not forget the glass of wine before dinner, the glass of wine during dinner, and the after-dinner drink (since we just called a cab).

Single-food or food-group diets are simply a complex way to control portions. If you control portions, then you will consume fewer calories. If you consume fewer calories, then you will lose weight. Surgery is the most radical of portion controls. Even if you have stretched your pouch a bit, or your stomach has grown, you still have a limited amount of space in which you can store foods you consume and you will lose weight. How much you lose is determined by the number of calories that you eat. From six months and beyond, you will still eat less although you might think you are eating a lot.

The simple recipes in this book contain ingredients that are good for you and your family, and some of them are personal favorites. We do not like single food diets for our patients, because more than anything we want our patients to have a variety; not because they deserve a lot of fine tasting food, but because variety in foods tends to have a variety of nutrients that a person with a smaller stomach needs. Single group diets are fine if you have a 40 or 50-ounce stomach, but not so good if your guts have been rearranged.

Where Do Patients Fail?

Patients fail because they fall into old eating and drinking habits—no time for breakfast, small lunch, lots of grazing in the afternoon, followed by a big dinner with dessert. It isn't intentional, it isn't planned, but the pattern is clear. Fast food places become their kitchens.

Dessert becomes a daily part of a meal instead of an occasional treat. Alcohol intake increases (remember, a beer a day will add ten pounds a year). Alcohol is absorbed, and so are its calories, almost anywhere in the gut, and so for no surgery blocks the absorption of alcohol. Then there are the soda drinkers—the pop goes down easy and the pounds start to come back on.

Is there a common theme to those patients who make and maintain their goal? How about the successful patients?

Every one of them eats breakfast, lunch, and dinner—every one. Some have a planned mid-afternoon snack and a light supper later, but every successful patient—that is, a patient who has a BMI of 24 or less, eats at least three meals a day. If you love food, then plan it and enjoy the planning. Figure out what you are going to eat on any given night as well as breakfast and lunch. It sure makes shopping easier. So that is why we have menu plans. We give them to you here—the menus for your meals—complete with calories, carbohydrate and protein counts to make certain you are getting enough food.

Menus and Recipes

Eggplant Parmesan

—recipe by a patient with RNY, loved by the lap-band patients and DS surgeons.

Café Sport in San Francisco is one of my favorite restaurants to have Eggplant Parmesan. In early July, I was there having dinner with my friend Robert Rabkin and his capable nurse, Barbara. That was the best Eggplant Parmesan I had ever tasted. In fact, the garlic was so great that the next morning my curtains melted from my garlic breath (good thing I didn't have to talk to patients that day). The next month I was in Mexico talking with Lee Grossbard, a lap-band surgeon who was celebrating the one-year anniversary of having his lap-band placed (and losing 120 pounds). I asked him what his first real food was after the lap-band surgery. He said, "Eggplant Parmesan." When I saw the recipe for Eggplant Parmesan in *Obesity Help Magazine* (for which I serve on the editorial board) I asked the author, Darcie Leigh, for the recipe.

Darcie Leigh is a well-known advocate in the weight-loss surgery world. She is not only a patient advocate; she is a patient. Darcie had her surgery from Dr. Andrei, an outstanding laparoscopic-bariatric surgeon in New Jersey. Over two years later, Darcie maintains a weight of 135 pounds on her 5-foot 8-inch frame, all while cooking for her family. Darcie is the mother of two. So my question was, "Do you cook any differently for your family than yourself?" The answer was "no." Being a good Italian girl, she did tell me that her mom's Eggplant Parmesan is better than her's. (Part of the price for getting these recipes was acknowledging this).

So, if you are wondering what successful patients love—as well as the surgeons of those patients (or in Lee's case, both a patient and a surgeon)—try this recipe. And one more tip: if you are ever eating dinner with a nice Italian family, the mother always makes it better than the daughter—never say otherwise.

Sample Menus & Meal Plans

Meal 1

	Calories	Protein	Carbs
Breakfast			
2 poached eggs	148	12	2
2 slices bacon	70	5	0
Snack			
1 stick string cheese	80	7	0
½ cup fresh fruit	30	1	7
Lunch			
1 cup Darcie's Chili & Cheese	205	18	9
Snack			
2 tbs Peanut Butter w/ rice cake	228	9	15
Dinner			
Chicken Parmesan	273	35	9
DAILY TOTALS	1034	87	42

Meal 2

	Calories	Protein	Carbs
Breakfast			
½ cup cottage cheese ½ cup mixed fruit	130	15	20
Snack			
2 oz Pork Rinds w/ ½ cup Salsa con Queso	100	10	4
Lunch			
3 oz chicken salad over lettuce	196	21	2
Snack			
2 oz mixed nuts	360	12	10
Dinner			
Grilled Salmon	311	22	6
DAILY TOTALS	1171	80	42

Meal 3

	Calories	Protein	Carbs
Breakfast			
1 egg cheese omelet	185	12	6
2 sausage links	180	6	1
Snack			
Turkey Pepperoni Chips	74	9	1
Lunch			
Crustless Low-Carb Quiche (spinach bacon & onion)	180	9	3
Snack			
4 oz low-fat yogurt	113	5	21
Dinner			
Grilled Beef Kabobs	281	27	3
DAILY TOTALS	1013	68	35

Meal 4

	Calories	Protein	Carbs
Breakfast			
1 egg omelet w/ 1 oz ham & 1 oz cheese	246	18	1
Snack			
Soy chips	110	7	15
Lunch			
4 oz cheeseburger (grilled or broiled no bread)	358	31	1
Snack			
2 sticks string cheese	160	14	0
Dinner			
Shrimp & Scallop Scampi	155	17	1
DAILY TOTALS	1029	87	18

Meal 5

	Calories	Protein	Carbs
Breakfast			
2 eggs scrambled	200	13	2
Snack			
Turkey Pepperoni Chips	74	9	1
Lunch			
Baked Eggplant Parmesan	220	11	19
Snack			
1 cup fresh fruit	60	1	13
Dinner			
BBQ Baby Back Ribs	472	40	4
DAILY TOTALS	1026	74	39

Recipes

for the Post-Op WLS Patient

Darcie's Chili & Cheese

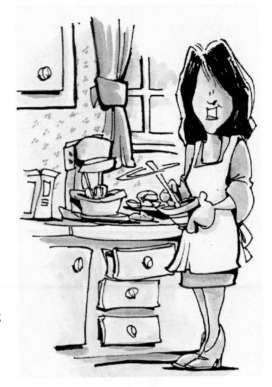

1 small onion chopped

1 stalk celery chopped

1 lb 93% lean ground beef

1 package chili seasoning mix

1 clove garlic

1 6-oz can tomato sauce

1 14-oz can white cannelloni beans

1 14-oz can diced tomatoes w/ juice

Shredded cheddar cheese

In saucepan over medium heat, sauté onion and celery until soft. Add ground beef and continue to sauté until beef is completely cooked. Drain excess fat. Add chili mix and stir to coat all the beef. Add the garlic, tomato sauce, beans, and diced tomatoes. Mix together well. Allow the chili to simmer for 15 minutes.

Top each 1-cup portion with 1 oz shredded cheese

Chicken Parmesan

Non-stick butter-flavored cooking spray

9 oz chicken cutlets pounded thin

1 cup marinara sauce

¼ cup grated Romano cheese

½ cup shredded mozzarella cheese

In large skillet over medium heat, spray pan with cooking spray and lightly brown cutlets on each side and place into a small casserole dish. Cover with marinara sauce and sprinkle with grated cheese. Then cover with shredded mozzarella. Bake for 20 minutes at 350°F.

Chicken Salad

6 oz cooked chicken, chopped

1/8 cup mayonnaise

1 tsp Dijon® mustard

1 tbs chopped onion

1 tbs chopped celery

salt & pepper

Mix all ingredients together well. Makes 2 servings.

Grilled Salmon

9 oz salmon

3 tbs butter melted

1 tbs chopped onion

2 tbs fresh lemon juice

1 tbs fresh herbs chopped (parsley & tarragon)

1 tsp white wine

salt & pepper

olive oil spray

Spray salmon with a spritz of olive oil on each side and season with salt and pepper. Grill fish until opaque.

In small skillet over medium heat, sauté onion in butter until soft. Add garlic & herbs. Stir in lemon juice with a fork until smooth. Spoon lemon/butter sauce over fish and serve. Makes 2 servings.

Turkey Pepperoni Chips

17 Turkey Pepperoni Slices

Separate slices onto a microwave safe dish and cook for 1 ½ minutes. Allow chips to cool. Makes 1 serving.

Crustless Low-Carb Quiche

4 eggs

1 cup half & half

¼ cup Bisquick®

¼ tsp nutmeg

1/8 tsp fresh ground pepper

½ cup frozen chopped spinach thawed and squeezed dry

4 slices crispy bacon (cooked in microwave)

1 cup shredded Swiss cheese

Preheat oven to 375°F. In 4-quart bowl beat eggs well for about 2 minutes. Add 1 cup half & half and continue beating for 1 minute. Stir in Bisquick, nutmeg, pepper, spinach, crumbled bacon and shredded Swiss cheese. Pour into a quiche plate and bake at 375°F for 35 minutes.

Grilled Beef Kabobs

½ lb lean bottom round beef cubes cut into 1 inch pieces

¼ cup Italian salad dressing

Place beef cubes in a zipper freezer bag and marinate for at least 1 hour. Place cubes onto skewers and grill for approximately 3 minutes on each side. (Try adding any veggies like onion, mushrooms, broccoli, or zucchini) Makes 2 servings.

Shrimp & Scallop Scampi

¾ pound shrimp

¾ pound scallops

2 tbs olive oil

2 tbs butter

2 tbs shallots finely chopped or thinly sliced scallions

1 tbs chopped fresh basil

1 tbs chopped fresh parsley

2 tbs lemon juice

¼ tsp salt

2 cloves garlic minced

Grated parmesan cheese to garnish if desired

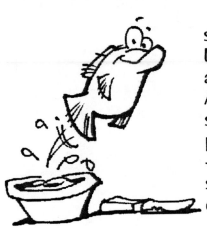

Heat oil and butter in a 10-inch skillet over medium heat. Add shallots, basil, parsley, lemon juice salt, and garlic. Blend well with a whisk. Add shrimp and scallops and cook stirring frequently until shrimp are pink and firm and scallops are opaque – about 3-4 minutes – and pour into a serving dish. Sprinkle with cheese if desired. Makes 6 servings.

Baked Eggplant Parmesan

1 medium eggplant – about 1 lb peeled and thinly sliced

2 eggs beaten with ¼ cup skim milk

2 cups Italian flavored breadcrumbs

32-oz jar marinara sauce

1 pound shredded part skim mozzarella

Olive oil in a sprayer

Fresh ground pepper

Preheat oven to 400°F and line 2 large cookie sheets with tin foil.

Dip thinly-sliced eggplant in egg/milk mixture and then dredge in breadcrumbs. Place each slice on baking sheets. Lightly spray with olive oil on both sides and bake for about 15-20 minutes until browned. Turn oven down to 350° F.

In a 2 quart rectangular baking dish, coat bottom with a layer of marinara sauce. Layer eggplant slices to slightly overlap and cover the bottom of the dish. Coat with another layer of sauce and sprinkle with grated mozzarella cheese and fresh ground pepper. Repeat all steps to create 2 more layers.

Bake at 350° for about ½ hour – cut into 15 servings

BBQ Baby Back Ribs

2 lbs baby back ribs
½ cup ketchup
½ tsp garlic powder
½ tsp onion powder
½ tsp seasoned salt
¼ cup Splenda®

Pre-heat oven to 400°

In a medium bowl mix ketchup, garlic powder, onion powder, seasoned salt and Splenda®. Coat ribs with one-half of the BBQ sauce. Line a baking tray with tin foil then roast ribs for 1 hour. Coat ribs with remaining BBQ sauce and roast for 30 minutes. Makes 6 servings.

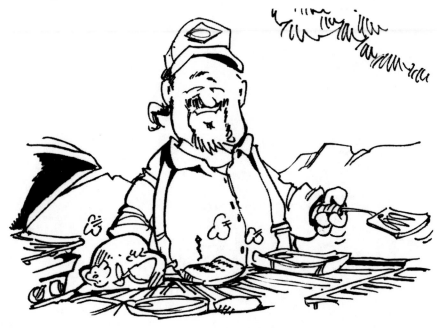

Part 5

Appendices

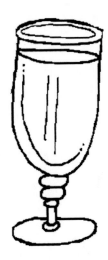

Appendix One

Liquids, Full Liquids, Purees

Sugar Free Clear Liquids

- apple Juice
- cranberry juice
- grape juice or white grape juice
- coffee or tea
- broth
- sugar-free gelatin
- sugar-free Kool-Aid® or Crystal Lite®
- sugar-free popsicles
- water
- IsoPure®

Sugar Filled Clear Liquids

- alcoholic beverages
- orange juice
- grapefruit juice
- Latte or Cappuccino
- cream soups
- regular Jell-O® or gelatin
- regular Kool-Aid®, lemonade
- regular popsicles
- Gatorade® or PowerAde®

Full Liquid Diet

All foods on the sugar-free clear liquid diet and the following:

- Cream of Wheat or Rice®

- Malt-o-meal®

- skim, 2% milk, or buttermilk (if lactose-intolerant consider lactaid tablets)

- Lactaid milk for lactose-intolerant

- soy milk

- plain yogurt (no fruits, nuts, seeds)

- Carnation Instant Breakfast® (sugar-free)

- Glucerna®

- soups—cream types

- diluted orange or grapefruit juice – unsweetened

Puree Diet

Food Group	Allowed Foods	Foods not Allowed
Liquids	See previous list of full liquids and clear liquids, these are all allowed	No Milkshakes. No alcohol. No Chocolate Milk. No pulpy juices (pulp in orange or grapefruit juice). No juice with seeds (tomato, V-8®, papaya). No sweetened juices. No hot chocolate.
Breads	An occasional soda cracker or Matzo for nausea	No breads. No cookies. No crackers
Cereal	Cream of Wheat®. Cream of Rice®. Malt-O-Meal®. Oatmeal. Do not put raisins, fruits, or sugar in these cereals. Be careful of some of these cereals if you have a lap-band as they might swell in the pouch	No cereal with nuts, seeds, or fruits, no Granola. No sugar-filled cereal. No Frosted Flakes®, No high-glycemic index cereals
Fruits	Puree all fruits, even bananas, which can stick in the stoma. Low-fiber fruits only: applesauce, apricots, melons, peaches, bananas. Canned fruits packed in water.	Avoid high-fiber fruits which will stick in your stoma, even pureed can cause significant problems. Avoid apples, avocados, blueberries, blackberries, huckleberries, dates, figs, grapefruits, lemons, limes, oranges, raspberries, strawberries. Avoid these in yogurts
Proteins	Tuna fish, shrimp, crab, any fish. Eggs in any form. Cottage cheese, tofu, peanut butter. Baby food meats. Puree lamb, pork, chicken, and duck. Boca® burgers. Cheeses of all kinds if they are SOFT. Yogurt – plain or flavored	Any fried meat, fish, chicken, or any fried food during this period. Beef is particularly difficult especially welldone. Avoid anything that doesn't blend well. Avoid Hard cheeses. No yogurt with fruit in the bottom.

Food Group	Allowed Foods	Foods not Allowed
Potatoes	Sweet potatoes - mashed potatoes, Pasta made from egg or spinach. Uncle Ben's® converted Rice.	No French Fries, no potato skins, no potato chips, no processed spaghetti, no processed lasagna, no corn chips.
Soups	Cream Soups, Consumé, broths, white clam chowder—puree the clams and potatoes. Puree chicken soups. Tomato is okay if there are no seeds.	No soups with corn, cabbage, cauliflower, broccoli, celery, or seeds. No bean soups. No onion soups. No soups with tomato skins.
Vegetables	Low-Fiber vegetables and puree vegetables, like those in baby food. Asparagus, beets, carrots, green beans, mushrooms, squash. Add bacon for flavor.	Avoid high-fiber vegetables. If you are in doubt, check to see if they have high-fiber content.
Dessert	An assortment of new high protein puddings is available. Sugar-free fudgesickles are there for certain patients (see comment below). Custards, sugar-free ice cream.	Regular sugar-filled ice cream, sherbet, gelatin, and popsicles. No pies. No cookies. No cakes. No pastries. No donuts.

Low-Fiber Vegetables

Low-fiber vegetables are acceptable during the puree diet. Patients who have the RNY, VBG, or lap-band may also eat these.

- asparagus
- beets
- carrots

- breen beans
- mushrooms
- summer squash

Vegetables With Fiber

Patients who have either the RNY, VBG, or lap-band should avoid high fiber foods in casseroles or soups. Patients with the DS can eat them but not during the puree diet phase.

* broccoli
* brussel sprouts
* cabbage
* cauliflower
* celery
* corn
* cucumbers
* dried beans
* onions

* peas
* pumpkin
* radishes
* rutabaga
* sauerkraut
* scallions
* tomatoes
* turnips
* winter squash

Use Your Blender Often During This Period

* Cut the food to the size of an eraser

* Put the portion in the blender

* Add liquid (vegetable stock, chicken stock) to just cover the blades

* Set it on puree, or high and blend until it is like a thick milkshake

* Measure out and store in Seal-a-meal bags or freezer bags in single unit portions

Moving from a Puree Diet to a Soft Diet

—slow and easy is the rule

As you move from the puree diet to a soft diet, you are in a transition phase. Every day you might try something new. You are testing your stomach. If something doesn't agree with you one day, don't despair. It takes time to get used to some foods. Some patients have cast-iron stomachs and can tolerate anything; other people find that their stomachs rebel after eating certain foods.

Foods that are typically hard to digest

- fried meats
- red meat (beef, pork – it really isn't the other white meat)
- game meats – venison, elk

Use your blender often during this period

- Cut the food to the size of an eraser

- Put the portion in the blender

- Add liquid (vegetable stock, chicken stock) to just cover the blades

- Set it on puree, or high and blend until it is like a thick milkshake

- Measure and store in Seal-a-meal® or freezer bags in single unit portions

Examples of low-glycemic index fruits and fruit juices

- oranges
- apples
- pears (including pears canned in pear juice)
- dried apricots
- peaches
- plums
- prunes
- grapefruits
- cherries
- prickly pears from arizona
- unsweetened grapefruit juice
- unsweetened apple juice
- unsweetened pineapple juice
- Raspberry Smoothie (product of Con Agra®)
- Agave Nectar® (light)

Examples of low-glycemic index vegetables

- sweet corn
- brown beans
- converted rice (Uncle Ben's® or Masterfoods®)
- butter beans
- split peas
- black beans
- lima beans
- navy beans/haricot
- pinto beans
- soy beans
- yams (peeled and boiled)
- chickpeas
- carrots
- lentils

Examples of low-glycemic index drinks

- Cappuccino
- Ultracal® with fiber (Mead Johnson)
- Glucerna® vanilla (Abbot Laboratories)
- Cappuccino
- Ultracal with fiber (Mead Johnson)
- Glucerna® vanilla (Abbot Laboratories)
- Nutrimeal® (Usana) – chocolate
- Choice DM®
- Resource Diabetic ®(Novartis Nutrition corp.)

Examples of low-glycemic index snacks (snacks-not meals)

- peanuts
- cashews
- peanut butter
- Apple-Cinnamon Snack Bar (Con Agra®)
- Peanut Butter and Chocolate Chip Snack Bar (Con Agra)
- Peanut Crunch Nutribar® (L.E.A.N. Life long)
- L.E.A.N® (Life long) Nutribar™, Chocolate Crunch
- Ironman PR Bar®, chocolate (PR Nutrition, San Diego, CA, USA)
- Ensure® Pudding, old-fashioned vanilla (Abbot Laboratories)
- hummus
- Twix Cookie Bar® (one of these only, not a bunch)

Examples of low-glycemic index breakfast choices

- eggs
- bacon
- cottage cheese
- yogurt (plain)
- hot cereal, apple and cinnamon (Con Agra®) – this will swell in your pouch, so be very careful.
- All-Bran® (Kellogg's) – this may swell, use caution

Examples of Glycemic Index for Certain Foods

Coca Cola	67	grapefruit juice, no sugar	48
Ocean Spray Cranberry	68	Sunkist orange	48
Wonder Bread (white)	77	frozen orange juice	57
Healthy Choice whole wheat	62	prunes, pitted	29
Nutty Natural	59	kidney beans	23
Kellogg's All Bran Cereal	38	lentils	28
Kellogg's Corn Flakes	92	spaghetti, wheat	64
rolled oats cereal	75	spaghetti, whole meal	32
Raisin Bran	61	Snicker's Bar	68
Special K	75	Power Bar, chocolate	58
sweet corn	60	russet potato, baked	85
Uncle Ben's Converted Rice	38	mashed potatoes, instant	97
ice cream	62	sweet potato	61
unsweetened apple juice	40	doughnut	76
yellow banana	51	apple	40
grapefruit half	25		

As you can see, some choices are better than others. The fruit is better than the juice, and whole grains are better than processed. Processed foods, strangely, tend to have a higher glycemic index than foods which are not processed. Again, the apple is better than the donut.

Protein Requirements

Protein requirements of patients who are morbidly obese are calculated upon lean body mass (what your weight is if your BMI was 24). The formula is 0.45 grams of protein required per pound for a BMI of 24.

This chart lists protein needs based on ideal body weight for your height and a BMI of 24. To determine the amount of protein required for sedentary activity, see the column for the surgery you had (or your length of common channel). For example, if you are 5-foot and 8-inches tall and had a proximal RNY bypass you will require 71 grams of protein per day. If you are 6 feet tall and had a DS, you will require 100 grams of protein per day.

| Height | Common Channel Size | | | |
	Normal Lap Band/VBG	400-500 cm Proximal RNY	200-400 cm Distal RNY	100 - 200 cm DS
5 foot	55 grams	55 grams	60 grams	70 grams
5'2"	58 grams	58 grams	65 grams	70 grams
5'4"	63 grams	63 grams	70 grams	75 grams
5'6"	66 grams	66 grams	72 grams	78 grams
5'8"	71 grams	71 grams	78 grams	85 grams
5'10"	75 grams	75 grams	82 grams	89 grams
6 foot	82.8 grams	82.8 grams	90 grams	100 grams

The length of the common channel is the key to protein requirements. Once the common channel is over 200 cm in length, the small bowel becomes very efficient at absorbing protein. For patients who develop severe protein malnutrition, lengthening the common channel by as little as 25 cm (about a foot) makes a substantial difference in their ability to absorb protein. It also can decrease diarrhea, increase absorption of bile, and will increase absorption of fat. Prior to undergoing surgery to lengthen the common channel, patients can be tried on pancreatic supplements. This allows more efficient digestion of protein and can often spare the patient a surgery.

Protein requirements increase with physical activity. The above numbers double for individuals who are in strength or endurance training. Following surgery, the requirements increase by twenty percent or more and can double for patients who suffer major burns.

Dietary intake is the key and modular protein supplementation may be required, especially in the early post-operative period when patients may have poor appetites or are intolerant of meats. Bioavailability of the protein is important, as some supplements contain essential amino acids that can be readily absorbed. Whey and egg white proteins are better absorbed than soy-based proteins. Gelatin-based proteins are not sufficient to sustain human metabolism and do not contain enough essential amino acids, so skip the Jell-O®.

Underweight	**BMI < 18.5 kg/m^2**
Normal Range	BMI 18.5-24.9 kg/m^2
Overweight	BMI 25- 30 kg/m^2
Class I obesity	BMI 30- 34.9 kg/m^2
Class II obesity (aka morbid obesity)	BMI 35 – 39.9 kg/m^2
Class III obesity	BMI 40 -49.9 kg/m^2
Class IV obesity	BMI > 50 kg/m^2

BMI Chart

Body Mass Index Chart

The following table lists the major BMIs. Find your height and locate your weight in the same row. If your weight is below the BMI of 35 then you are not eligible for most weight loss surgery. If your BMI is more than 40 then you are eligible for weight loss surgery.

Height in inches	BMI of 25	BMI of 30	BMI of 35	BMI of 40	BMI of 45	BMI of 50
4' 10"	120 lbs.	144 lbs.	167 lbs.	191 lbs.	215 lbs.	239 lbs.
4' 11"	124	14	174	198	223	248
5' 0"	128	153	179	205	230	256
5' 1"	132	159	185	212	238	265
5' 2"	137	164	191	219	246	273
5' 3"	141	169	198	226	254	282
5' 4'"	146	175	204	233	262	291
5' 5"	150	181	211	241	271	301
5' 6"	155	186	217	248	279	310
5' 7"	160	192	224	256	288	320
5' 8"	164	197	230	263	296	329
5' 9"	169	203	237	271	305	338
5' 10"	174	209	244	279	313	348
5' 11"	179	215	251	287	322	358
6' 0"	185	222	259	295	332	369
6' 1"	190	228	265	303	341	379
6' 2"	195	233	272	311	350	389
6' 3"	200	240	280	320	360	400
6' 4"	206	247	288	329	370	411

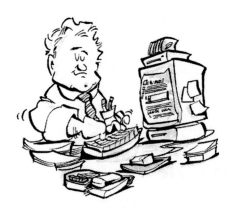

Appendix Two

Dear Doctor...

What Your Doctor Needs To Know

Overweight people are not the only ones who need information about weight loss surgery. Sometimes doctors also need information so that they can help their patients make the right decisions about weight loss surgery or help them with the aftercare.

Are you a doctor with a patient who is considering weight loss surgery? Has a patient asked for your opinion or a referral for a bariatric surgeon? Do you have a patient who has had weight loss surgery and has now come to you for after-care? There are several things you need to know about weight loss surgery so you can help your patient either make the right choice about the surgery, or to heal quickly and achieve his or her weight loss goal after the surgery.

As you know, not all weight loss surgeries are alike. In medical school, you may have heard horror stories about the jejuno-ileal bypass, or how "stomach stapling" didn't really work. Now you are reading about celebrities, and even politicians, who have had the procedures! Weight loss surgery has changed and advanced, but the success does not depend entirely on the type of surgery that is done—often it is the aftercare. Sometimes, the most important step you can provide for the weight loss surgery patient is the aftercare.

Weight loss surgery does work, but patients often need more follow-up care than many bariatric surgeons can give. As a result, the burden may fall on you, the family doctor, to help organize and manage the whole group of tests, post op follow-ups, and various complaints that your patient will have.

Who Should You Refer to a Bariatric Surgeon?

Which patients should you refer to a bariatric surgeon and when? The answer lies in the NIH guidelines: those patients who have a BMI of 35 with or without co-morbidities or those with a BMI of 40 with no co-morbidities. This might look like a large group of patients but you can narrow it down. The ones to refer are those that are unlikely to benefit from any long-lasting solution besides weight loss surgery.

The ones to refer are those that are unlikely to benefit from any long-lasting solution besides weight loss surgery.

Often the first patients a physician refers to a surgeon are patients who are "super morbidly obese." Usually these patients are in the 500-pound club. While these patients should be referred, remember that these patients are the ones who have suffered the most from the ravages of morbid obesity and will be the most challenging for the surgeon and the anesthesiologist. I had a cardiologist refer a patient with severe heart disease who weighed 400 pounds. He died before he came to the operating room. Had that patient been referred five years earlier when he weighed 300 pounds, I often wonder—would he be alive today? So, when considering referral of patients to the bariatric surgeon, remember that the NIH criteria are a good place to start.

Prepare Your Patients for Success

Many insurance companies require a physician-supervised weight loss program of at least six months. This must be completed within two years of the referral for surgery. As you are talking to your patient about weight loss, document his or her weight and begin the patient on a program for weight loss right away. Prescription drugs for weight loss are not necessary, although some patients do find these helpful. Nevertheless, the best programs involve patient nutritional classes, some counseling, and weekly weigh-ins. You don't have to see the patient weekly, but having him come to the office and weigh on your scale is helpful to the patient.

Components of a good weight loss program:

- Nutritional classes or lectures
- Weekly or at least every other week, weigh-in. Calculate BMI.
- A diet plan (document attendance at Weight Watchers, for example)
- Check yearly post op labs blood levels at the start
- Physical therapy consult for planning an exercise program—safe stretching
- Water aerobics classes for patients with joint problems
- Teach the patient to take his or her pulse and set goals for heart rate with exercise
- Stress test, if needed

Prescriptions are not necessary, but if medication is prescribed, be sure to document any side effects

---

Some physicians find "package" plans, such as Opti-fast, to be helpful. However, these are not necessary. Most insurance companies want to know that the patient, under the care of his primary care physician, has made an effort at weight loss. Hopefully this will be successful and the patient will keep the weight off, rendering the surgery unnecessary—but, as per the consensus statement from the NIH, this is unlikely. Nevertheless, a small percent of patients will lose enough weight that surgery is not necessary.

Many diet plans and programs are available, and a lot of groups are designed to help support the patient. There are multiple types of plans, but insurance companies do not care if a patient has been to Weight-Watchers—what they want is physician supervision and intervention. While the patient is working with you, adjuncts, such as Weight-Watchers, are always helpful, as the more information a patients can obtain, the better prepared they will be. There is no magic diet, just as there is no magic food. Moderation in all things, including moderation, is the key—or, eat less, move more. The reason single-food diets, or single food-type diets (Atkins) work well is that people eat multiple foods, not just one.

There is no magic diet, just as there is no magic food.

Physical activity is the key to success in any weight loss program, and this is one place where you can help your patients. A physical therapist can teach them to "warm up" and stretch, before starting a walking or water aerobics program. This is very helpful in preventing early injuries. Patients should learn to take their own pulse, or they should purchase one of those cute devices to check their pulse while exercising and after. Give your patient targets for pulse and heart rates, and also give them warnings.

Certainly all patients will benefit from vitamins and supplements (such as calcium), as the typical "American" diet seems to be lacking in many vitamins and minerals. It is a good idea to have patients start out with these supplements.

Preparing the Referral Letter

The referral letter from you to the insurance company is important. If your letter to the insurance company documents that the patient has been under your supervision for at least six months, you are providing the key to insurance approval. Sometimes bariatric surgeons have long wait-times so you can use this time to have patients on a supervised diet/weight loss program. However, a letter is often not enough. Many insurance companies also want chart notes. Having a chart note that says they are obese and should lose weight will not be enough to convince an insurance company that your patient has been under a "physician-supervised" program. Notes are proof that the patient has been under your supervision for weight loss, that they have seen a nutritionist or dietician, and that they are being supervised in a manner that shows their primary care doctor has been involved. Putting together a program for all your obese patients, including classes and activities, is a great thing to offer not only morbidly obese patients but others who want to lose a few pounds before the swimsuit season.

Learn About Your Bariatric Surgeon

Some bariatric surgeons offer one type of surgery, and some another. Some will be on the same insurance plans as your patients and some will not. Ask a couple of these bariatric surgeons to come to your office or to the hospital and to give a talk to your patients about bariatric surgery. It is a good way to learn the types of surgery they perform and a little about their office procedures. Some bariatric surgeons prefer to follow every laboratory value of the patient and some will quickly turn the task over to you. Either way, stay in the loop so you know what is happening with your patients. It will provide you with bariatric surgeon referral choices, and you will learn what the surgeon expects your role to be. If your patients are going out of state for weight loss surgery, ask the surgeon to call you so you can create a game plan for the patient. That way both you and the patient will know what to expect.

Vena Cava Filters

Some patients, knowing that pulmonary embolism is the most common cause of death, will request that a filter be placed in their Inferior Vena Cava. These filters are not without morbidity risks and can cause permanent problems for a patient, especially if their IVC clots off. There are some "removable" filters, which might be an option, although some of these filters have their own associated morbidity. This is not something a patient should decide. You should discuss it with the hematologist and the surgeon. While there are some general guidelines for placement, there are no absolutes.

> ## Consider a pre-operative Vena Cava filter if:
> - the patient has had a pulmonary embolus before
> - the patient has had DVT while on Coumadin or Heparin
> - the patient has an allergy to heparin

Medicines Before and After Surgery

After weight loss surgery, a patient's reaction to medication may be different than it was before surgery. It is important to know how a patient will react after the guts are rearranged. Some medications cannot be swallowed well after a RNY or lap-band (particularly large pills). Some medications, especially time-released, are not absorbed as well. Patients who had a distal bypass should not be on a time-released medication. Go through the list of medications with your patient—if there are liquid forms available, or chewable forms, then change to those.

> ## After the guts are rearranged:
> - convert time-release medicines to regular, non-time released forms
> - find chewable or liquid forms of medicines
> - determine if the medicines can be crushed and retain their effectiveness

Some medications clearly need to be stopped before surgery, such as blood thinners (Coumadin, Plavix, aspirin), and may need to be substituted with other medications. Other medicines that should be stopped include birth control pills and hormone replacement therapy, as the incidence of deep venous thrombosis with these medicines is increased. The statins (Lipitor, Pravachol, etc) have been associated with a small, but real, incidence of rhabdomyalysis after surgery, so these medications should be stopped at least one week prior to surgery.

> **Stop these medicines before surgery:**
> - aspirin, Plavix, coumadin
> - Lipitor, Pravachol, and other statins
> - estrogens, hormone replacement therapy, birth control pills

Oral hypoglycemic medications should be stopped the day before surgery and should not be started until after surgery. They should be restarted only if the patient develops high blood sugars. Patients cannot consume the same quantities of calories after surgery so their blood sugar will drop, and many will not need these medicines following surgery. Insulin requirements will also decrease, and these patients need to be monitored carefully and doses adjusted accordingly.

Continue beta-blockers throughout the hospital stay. If patients don't need these for blood pressure control, then wean them off carefully.

Most patients will come home from the hospital with excess fluid in their extremities. This is quite normal. While some diuretics are helpful in mobilizing these fluids, this is short-term and the patient should be encouraged to continue with protein drinks and supplements. The colloidal action of protein will help to mobilize the fluid. Generally it will only take a few days of diuretics.

Anti-hypertensive drugs are tricky in the post-operative period. Generally, a patent's blood pressure decreases in the initial post-operative period only to rise a bit when they return home. These patients may need to monitor their own blood pressure, or come to the office for weekly visits with the nurse to monitor their blood pressure and adjust medication. While they may not need medication in the first couple of weeks, their high blood pressure hasn't gone away. It has just been moderated a bit from surgery, and they will need their usual dose again. Most bariatric surgeons note that real changes in blood pressure medications occur after the first forty pounds are lost.

Immediate post-op
- monitor blood glucose, do not start oral hypoglycemics
- watch blood pressure levels

What Consultants Should You Have On Your Team?

The consultant you will need more than any other is probably a gastroenterologist. RNY or other patients may need dilation of their stomas, anastomosis, or stomachs. In addition, many weight loss surgery patients develop problems with diarrhea or constipation. These patients can be a challenge. They often have common GI problems that need to be addressed. RNY-gastric bypass patients cannot have parts of their GI tract evaluated. The gastroenterologist cannot maneuver the endoscope into the lower stomach or the duodenum (unless it is a very short proximal limb and you have a very talented gastroenterologist). This means that ERCP will be impossible to get into patients who have had RNY, BPD, or the DS surgery. With DS patients, you can scope the entire stomach, as well as the post pyloric duodenum—but a gastroenterologist cannot get to that part of the duodenum necessary to perform an ERCP. Patients who have the lap-band or the VBG have their entire GI tract available for endoscopy.

If the surgeon did not remove the gallbladder at the time of weight loss surgery, then it is important to watch for signs and symptoms of cholecystitis. Large changes in weight, as happens with any patient who diets, can precipitate gallstones. So many patients are at risk for cholecystitis. Remember, unless your patient had the lap-band or the VBG, the gastroenterologist cannot do an ERCP. If they develop gallstones, make certain the gallbladder is removed before the stones migrate down the duct. Any qualified surgeon can do gallbladder removal laparoscopically even if your patient had an "open" gastric bypass surgery.

Many obese patients have sleep apnea, and as they lose weight, their sleep apnea needs to be reevaluated. No patient is happier than one who gets rid of a CPAP machine. A pulmonologist must be involved with the patient to facilitate this.

Early Nausea and Vomiting

Early nausea and vomiting are common with post-operative patients. Often it is because they overeat (really, their eyes are bigger than their stomachs—in fact, their mouths hold more than their stomachs—talk about inverse biology). Visualizing a shot glass, or three shot glasses (depending on the size of the pouch or stomach), sometimes helps patients learn to measure food twice, eat once, and vomit never.

Some foods are tolerated one day and not tolerated the next. One day tuna can be the greatest thing, the next day it comes back up. This is a period of adjustment for the stomach and the patient. If vomiting continues, patients need to stop eating entirely and take a teaspoon of liquid (water is preferred) every five minutes while awake. That will keep them hydrated without stretching their stomach and inducing vomiting. They can slowly progress from here. Vomiting is the enemy in early weight loss surgery patients. It can cause a slip of the lap-band, can disrupt staples, and can even cause a rupture of the esophagus (Boerhaave's syndrome). Fortunately, those complications are rare, but avoiding vomiting is important.

Bowel obstruction is always a concern in any post-operative patient.

Patients who have diabetes often have a gastroparesis and will need to be on Reglan before meals and at bedtime.

Stomal stenosis cannot be diagnosed with an upper GI, but can be diagnosed with endoscopy and treated at the same time. Often if they have this stenosis, they will need several dilations. A stenosis can also occur in the mid-body of the stomach in patients who have had the duodenal switch. So, keep your gastroenterologist's number handy.

If a patient continues vomiting, he needs to be hospitalized and made n.p.o., given some round the clock medication (Zofran), and placed on intravenous fluids. Remember to give your patients Thiamin, as well as multivitamins, in the intravenous fluids to avoid Vitamin B deficiency. While the patient is hospitalized, you can strictly regulate his intake (giving 60 cc per hour per OS maximum) and if the nausea disappears with such regulation, then reinforce the rule about not out-eating the pouch.

Bowel obstruction is always a concern in any post-operative patient. Pain, nausea and vomiting may mean emergency surgery. These patients should be admitted and have appropriate x-rays taken (CT of the abdomen and pelvis, as well as three views of the abdomen). Remember, if the patient had some bowel bypassed, there will be unopacified bowel on the CT scan, and that might be mistaken for an abscess—so communicate that with the radiologist.

Checking Laboratory Values

In medical school, we were taught that our bodies store enough B12 to last a couple of years—turns out that isn't quite the case. Patients who have a Roux-en-Y gastric bypass can become deficient in B12 within four months. Iron levels can also decrease quickly, so we recommend a CBC at three months and again at six months. Order other tests based on those results. B12 levels can be checked at six months. Some patient just love getting B12 shots—although the sublingual from is equally effective. Therapy should be based on B12 levels and response, and not just a set schedule.

Pre-menopausal women should take Chromagen Forte or some type of iron. Be sure it is not mixed with calcium. Iron supplementation is not needed for all patients and some forms of iron will cause the stomach to be quite upset, so if the patient takes some iron and vomits, switch to a type of iron she can tolerate. Some patients may even require iron given intravenously or intramuscularly, as that is the only way they will absorb the iron.

Anemia is not "normal" for weight loss surgery patients, and demands a work-up. Don't assume that surgery is the cause of iron or B12 deficiency. Do a work-up to rule out bone marrow suppression, ongoing blood loss from the GI tract, as well as premature destruction of red blood cells.

Distal bypass patients frequently need to have vitamin K levels monitored as a protime (although clearly other things can effect protime). If they are getting bruised a bit, it may be vitamin K related.

Alkaline phosphatase rises not because of the liver enzymes component, but because bone is being used as a source of calcium. Calcium replacement is needed in almost all patients, but especially in distal bypass patients. Often up to

2000 grams per day in divided doses is needed to get the alkaline phosphatase or the parathyroid hormone to normal levels.

Don't be alarmed if the total cholesterol is low, the HDL levels are also low, while VLDL is high. There is no evidence this is a problem. However, with either an increase in fish consumption, flaxseed oil, or the pill form of omega 3 fatty acids, the HDL level can rise. Part of your job is to teach patients about good food—and that fish is good for them.

Vitamin B levels can fall to low levels, especially in patients who have a lot of vomiting. This is easy to correct, but worthwhile remembering when admitting a patient for dehydration. Some cases of Weneicke-Korsakoff encephalopathy have been reported so adding multivitamins to the IV solution for patients who are dehydrated is useful, as is giving thiamin.

Part of your job is to teach patients about good food–and that fish is good for them.

All liver enzymes rise in response to protein starvation during the time patients are getting most of their calories from carbohydrates. NASH (Non-alcoholic Steatohepatitis) is common among obese patients, and can lead to cirrhosis. Prompt treatment with protein is helpful. If a patient has severe protein-calorie malnutrition, they can develop an elevation of liver enzymes. Some bariatric surgeons routinely biopsy all livers for NASH—while this makes for interesting articles, it is not needed. If your patient develops elevated liver enzymes, have your gastroenterologist intervene.

Another symptom of mild protein malnutrition is light-headedness. This is often cured by having patients supplement their diet with protein shakes. While food is the best source, protein shakes are good. Those made of egg whites or whey are better than those of soy products. Some protein-deficient patients will develop leg edema, become listless, and have nausea. Occasionally these patients need pancreatic enzymes added to their meals, and sometimes they need to have TPN or a feeding tube to get them through.

Labs drawn at six months post surgery:

- CBC
- B12 levels
- pre-albumin
- complete metabolic panel
- hepatic function panel

Weight loss surgery patients are some of the most pleasurable patients to have. You will see dramatic weight loss and improvement in co-morbidities (sleep apnea, hypertension, diabetes, and joint problems). If you have several weight loss patients in your practice, and are getting more, I would encourage you to form a support group for them. You will enjoy watching them go through the weight loss process and members of the group will be a great help and encouragement to each other.

Chart information

Physicians referring patients to a weight loss surgeon are often asked to prescribe for the patient six months of a physcian-supervised diet. The insurance companies will ask for your chart notes. This template is an example of the information the chart notes should contain. Please be certain to see your patient at least two times per month during this period.

Patient Chart

PatientName:_____Date_____

Age _____ Height _____ Weight _____BMI _____

Goal at BMI of 24 _____B/P _____ Pulse _____

Diet Plan Discussed:

(a)   Low-Carbohydrate (Atkins)

(b)   Mayo Clinic Diet

(c)   Ornish (low-fat)

(d)   Weight Watchers (point system)

Date patient started diet _____ Weight at start of diet _____

Weight loss on diet _____ Weight gain since starting diet _____

Nutritionist/Dietician consultation (enter date) _____

Morbid Obesity [ICD-9 278.01] related co-morbidities of this patient:

Hypertension [ICD-9 401.1]

    Improved with diet _____ Condition has worsened _____

Diabetes Mellitus controlled [250.0] _____poorly controlled [250.2]_____

    Improved with diet _____ Condition has worsened _____

Sleep apnea [780.51]   Requires CPAP [780.54]

    Improved with diet _____ Condition has worsened_____

Cardiovascular disease [429.2]

Congestive heart failure [428.0]

Osteoarthritis [715.0]

Medications taken for above conditions

New medications required for above conditions

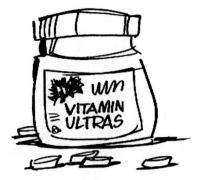

Appendix Three

Vitamins

During weight loss surgery, the surgeon rearranges the guts in order to change the genetic predisposition of a patient so they can go from being obese to being thin. While we cannot change the environmental factors in the patient's life that caused him or her to be obese, we can re-route the system a bit to aid the patient with weight loss. As a result, a number of vitamins and minerals will need supplementation. This chapter provides an A-Z guide for patients and their primary care physicians on what supplements are needed for the different types of surgery, and how to check for deficiencies.

Theme of All Weight Loss Surgeries...

Deficiencies—easy to prevent, not easy to treat!

No matter which weight loss surgery you have, preventing a deficiency is fairly simple: in most cases it simply involves taking a vitamin, and in some other cases it may involve taking shots (not Tequila, either). Treating a deficiency is not easy and is more complex than just taking a vitamin. No matter which weight loss surgery you have, you should take supplements. If you don't take them, you can become very sick, you can become permanently disabled, and you can die.

Iron Deficiency

Iron is absorbed primarily in the duodenum but it is also absorbed in the small bowel. Some patients with duodenal switch, therefore, will have no problem with iron levels, but this is variable. RNY gastric bypass patients are particularly prone to iron malabsorption. Some studies have suggested that menstruating women should take iron twice a day, as either ferrous sulfate or ferrous gluconate (300-350 mg per day). Ferrous fumarate, used in Chromagen® Forte Capsules, is an organic iron complex which has the highest elemental iron content of any hematinic salt - 33%. This compares with 20% for ferrous sulfate (heptahydrate) and 13% for ferrous gluconate.[1,2] Chromagen® Forte contains 151 mg of elemental iron. While this still will not completely prevent iron deficiency, it greatly reduces the number of patients who will have problems with it.

Iron-containing foods include meats, poultry, oysters, rusty nails, and dark leafy vegetables.

Recommended tests

Complete Blood Count (CBC) every six months first two years, then yearly thereafter. If anemia is found then additional tests include serum ferritin. Bone marrow examination is the most specific, but serum ferritin levels are proportional to marrow iron and inversely proportional to transferrin levels. Iron deficiencies, and decreased stores, are associated with ferritin levels below 15ng/mL in men, and 10ng/mL in women. Values between 15ng/mL and 100ng/mL can indicate deficiency in patients with an inflammatory process. Inflammation can lead to falsely high ferritin levels. In patients who have inflammatory process that is ongoing, treatment with iron, and the response to the therapy, may be the best diagnostic approach, short of bone marrow stains.

Serum iron and binding capacity are often ordered at the same time, and they may confirm an inadequate iron store. Elevated red cell distribution width (seen on CBC) may be helpful in monitoring response to therapy, but is inadequate to determine iron deficiency.

Treatment with Rusty Nails

Treatment of iron deficiency can be complicated with post-operative patients. Oral iron is inexpensive, and can be tried for several months. Iron absorption is aided with the addition of vitamin C, and is mildly inhibited with calcium. The addition of 500 mg of vitamin C with the iron increases iron absorption. But with many patients, oral intake will not produce a fast enough response. Sometimes iron must be taken through shots (intramuscular or intravenous). These patients should be watched carefully to avoid iron overload. The body becomes very efficient at absorbing iron if it is deficient.

Vitamin B Deficiencies

Vitamin B1 (Thiamin) Deficiency

While this is readily available in multivitamins, deficiency of this simple vitamin can cause severe neurologic problems (Wernicke's syndrome). Early symptoms of Thiamin deficiency can be headaches, anorexia, weakness, edema, lowered blood pressure, low body temperature, nausea, and muscle aches and pains. Patients who have persistent vomiting, or difficulty eating, or those rare patients who become anorectic, can develop severe syndromes such as Wernicke's. Wernicke's is manifested as depression, inability to concentrate or to learn, hallucinations, confabulation (making up stories unintentionally—unlike fishermen), and ultimately by difficulty walking (gait) and even dementia. Ultimately patients can also develop Beriberi, heart failure and peripheral edema.

Tests for Vitamin B1 levels are expensive and time-consuming, but treatment is quite simple. If a patient is having difficulty with nausea and anorexia, thiamine is available as a pill or in injectable forms. Just as we do not give glucose without thiamin for alcoholic patients, giving glucose without thiamin for patients who have been vomiting and may malabsorb can induce a Wernicke's.

Since the vitamin is water-soluble, no toxic effects have been reported in humans.

Vitamin B12 (Cobalamin)

When I was a young man, it was a popular thing for patients to go see the doctor for their monthly B12 injection to give them energy. They probably didn't need it, but a pat on the back by our small-town physician and a shot was something that made a lot of them feel pretty good. B12 deficiency in patients who have had weight loss surgery can be a real issue, however, and one that is easy to prevent.

While the liver stores a lot of B12, the previous estimate that patients have adequate stores for a year or longer are probably incorrect. Most B12 deficiency is manifested in weight loss patients within about three months. B12 is a necessary vitamin to build healthy blood cells, and without it anemia will occur. B12 is not absorbed unless it is combined with a factor in the stomach called "intrinsic factor," hence, gastric bypass patients have a propensity to develop this deficiency.

Most B12 deficiency is manifested in weight loss patients within about three months.

Symptoms are manifested by weakness, fatigue, and shortness of breath, all of which are secondary to the anemia. Other signs include a sore tongue, lack of taste, some heartburn, numbness, hair loss, impotence, irritability and memory disturbances. Depression is a common manifestation of this. Jaundice can also occur with B12 deficiency. Blood cells are broken down, but unable to be made, so one of the breakdown products, bilirubin, makes you yellow. The problem with jaundice is that it is so hard to find clothes to match the yellow color.

Treatment can yield impressive results with a single injection of 100μg after 24 hours. Before beginning therapy, however, it is important to confirm the diagnosis. The patient should be followed with a hemoglobin, hematocrit, erythrocyte, and reticulocyte count.

Once the clinical symptoms have improved and the blood count is returning to normal, a monthly maintenance dose of 100 to 200 mcg will be sufficient to maintain the patient. Patients who have this need to have lifelong therapy, while they can store the drug for a while, they need to understand that this is something they will need for the rest of their life.

The Schilling test reflects absorption of B12. Serum B12 can be checked directly which correlates with body stores. A serum level of less than 140 pg/mL is always associated with low body stores; however, this can be altered if the patient has a protein deficiency or a folate deficiency. Hence, with ordering a serum B12 level we recommend a serum methylmalonic acid and total homocysteine level. The Schilling test is rarely, if ever, used today. Often we use B12 levels and serum methylmalonic acid levels and serum homocystine levels instead.

Vitamin B6 deficiency: increased homocysteine, and decreased d-cystathionine. Folate deficiency will show increased homocysteine, and decreased 2-methyl citric acid. Cobalamin (B12) deficiency will show increased homocysteine and increased methylmalonic acid.

Vitamin B6

This is a complicated vitamin that is produced in the upper intestine, and malabsorption is a known cause for its deficiency. Too much of the vitamin can lead to a neuropathy, so it is one of those where too much can be a bad thing. Deficiency of this vitamin is also with non-specific symptoms such as seborrhea-like lesions around the eyes, nose, mouth; glossitis; hypochromic anemia; peripheral neuritis. Other symptoms such as nausea and vomiting, dizziness and insomnia have been described. One can order a Vitamin B6 level, although replacement therapy with a B complex, if this is suspected, is fairly simple. RBC folate levels are very helpful.

Folate

Ever notice that most of these B vitamins have some of the same symptoms? Anorexia, nausea, diarrhea, mouth ulcers, hair loss, fatigue, a sore tongue, and anemia are all signs of folate deficiency. Folate deficiency is a real problem for women who wish to become pregnant, as a class of birth defects, known as neural tube defects, is associated with folate deficiency (spina bifida type). Again, this is something that is easy to prevent. Serum homocysteine (but not methylmalonic acid) levels are elevated in folate deficiency.

Fat-Soluble Vitamins A, D, E, K

–Polar Bears and Anti-Oxidants

This class of vitamins may be low in patients who have had either a distal RNY or duodenal switch surgery. However these vitamins are stored in the body and toxic overdose can occur. Some is good, but more is not better. Polar bear liver (seriously) has high concentrations of Vitamin A, so much so that cases of toxicity have been reported from eating their liver. I don't know if you add Fava beans what would happen.

Vitamin A is needed for the eye, but lately importance has been placed on the carotene portion of Vitamin A, and its use as an anti-oxidant to prevent chronic diseases. But eye changes have been well studied, and they go from poor dark adaptation to scarring and softening of the cornea. There is also some evidence that Vitamin A facilitates wound healing, especially in patients who use steroids. Certain additives in food can decrease absorption of vitamin A, such as the cholestyramine (which some patients are taking for a bile salt diarrhea), mineral oil, and the popular ingredient Olestra. Vitamin A levels may be ordered directly and they take a lab a couple of weeks, usually, to return. One fellow who had a duodenal switch didn't take his vitamins very often, and woke up one morning blind. Fortunately, it reversed but this is not always the case. Take your vitamins, and make sure your levels are checked regularly.

Vitamin D deficiency has been noted in surgical residents, people who live in northern climates, and many people during the wintertime. Vitamin D is an essential component in calcium metabolism. There has been some thought that seasonal affective disorder (SAD) may be related to vitamin D deficiency. This can be examined directly with the 1, 25-Dihydroxyvitamin D assays. Serum alkaline phosphatase levels become elevated in vitamin D deficiency, although this is a relatively non-specific test, in patients who have had gastric bypass this is one of the factors which needs to be examined. The main concern is bone loss (or demineralization) over time. Bones can lose calcium, while the body maintains a normal serum calcium level, and patients can develop osteoporosis. So, again, some patients think that because their blood level of calcium is "normal" that they are taking enough calcium supplements, or are getting enough from their diet—a very dangerous and incorrect assumption. Again, the deficiency is easy to prevent, but once manifested is difficult to treat.

Vitamin E is one of those vitamins that has been looking for a reason to exist. I remember when it was supposed to enhance your sex life, then it was supposed to be good for the heart, then it fought cancer. Well, it might do all of those things, but in patients with distal bypass or the DS, this is a vitamin that might be a bit low. Some people have a genetic inability to transfer vitamin E to tissues, and these individuals have some neurologic problems. Vitamin E is thought to have great anti-oxidant properties, and have beneficial effects with a wide range of diseases. Since Vitamin E is a catch-all for "tocopherols" it may be that we will have more specific information about this class of vitamin as time goes on. Suffice it to say, there are a lot of good reasons to take this vitamin. There is no simple assay to measure it. Again, too many fat-soluble vitamins can be toxic. Do not take more unless you are under a physician's instruction and care.

The fat soluble vitamins are often sold in one pill called, strangely enough, ADEK

Vitamin K is the last of the fat-soluble vitamins, and is the deficiency that most patients manifest. Patients will have easy bruising and problems with their blood clotting (ever wondered why when you shaved there was blood in the bathroom?). Most often patients will come into my office and show me bruises on their arms and legs and wonder why they are having them. Vitamin K is a necessary component of the clotting mechanism, and checking a prothrombin time (PT or protime) is an easy way to tell if there is a deficiency.

The fat-soluble vitamins are often sold in one pill called, strangely enough, ADEK—and patients who have had a distal bypass or a DS sometimes need to take these in addition to a regular multivitamin.

Calcium

–Strong Bones, Teeth, and Skull

Calcium is required in a lot of complex biochemical reactions, it is required in your bones, and it is not present in a lot of foods. Hence, most patients who have undergone some weight loss surgery should be on calcium supplementation. Since calcium isn't absorbed that well, and since there is loss of calcium in the urine and in the stool, this is one of the most common deficiencies physicians see in patients. Most weight loss surgery patients are on high-protein diets, and high-protein intake causes an increase in calcium in the urine. So the best way to have a calcium deficiency is to have a high-protein diet without supplementation of calcium, have had weight loss surgery so you cannot take in a lot of calcium, develop lactose intolerance so you lose your major source of calcium, and be on a diuretic that causes an increase in calcium in the urine—in other words—the average post-op bariatric patient. To differentiate between liver and bones get a GGTP level. If the GGTP is normal, the alkaline phosphatase is most likely from bones, if it is high then consider a more extensive work up of the liver.

We highly recommend that patients who undergo weight loss surgery have bone density measurements.

Foods that contain calcium include milk (about 280 to 300 mg of calcium per cup), cheese, (200-280 mg. of calcium per ounce), spinach (1 cup is about 240 mg of calcium—and you get great looking forearms), sardines, and salmon.

Serum calcium levels can be normal, when the body is removing calcium from bones to keep blood levels normal. Alkaline phosphatase levels can be elevated if calcium is being leached from the bones, although this is somewhat non-specific. We highly recommend that patients who undergo weight loss surgery have bone density measurements, and that these be followed by the primary care physician. The DEXA test (okay, for those of you who are nerds this would be the dual-energy absorptiometry) is the most common one used today.

There are a few things to remember: first, calcium citrate is better absorbed than calcium carbonate. Second, calcium supplements should not be taken at the same time as iron—which makes me wonder why some companies put iron and calcium in the same pill. In fact, calcium can interfere with a number of other medications, and should simply be taken by itself, and not with any other medicines (atenolol, tetracyclines, aspirin, etc.). Most bariatric surgeons recommend far more calcium than the upper limit set by most standards—the upper limit being 1200 mg/d while most bariatric surgeons recommend 1800 to 2000 mg/d.

Stones, Bones, and Abdominal Moans

Okay—that is an old saying about hyperparathyroidism, but I love how it flows out of my mouth so much, I thought I would use this as an excuse to talk about calcium oxalate stones. The jejuno-ileal bypass patients had a high incidence of kidney stones made from calcium oxalate. Patients who have a distal bypass, or have a duodenal switch, also have malabsorption of fat and can have increased absorption of oxalate, leading to calcium oxalate stones. To counter this, the more calcium they take, the more sodium will combine with oxalate in the gut, and the less likely they will have kidney stones. Of course, there are many other types of kidney stones and the proper way to work up kidney stones is to have the stones analyzed and then determine the cause. Nevertheless, taking calcium is a good thing for patients who have undergone the duodenal switch.

Magnesium and Phosphorus

While these should be checked yearly, with simple blood tests, there is no evidence that weight loss surgery causes a problem with their levels, nor is there evidence to consider supplementation of these minerals. Diarrhea can cause loss of magnesium, so with some distal bypass patients a magnesium level should be checked if they are having diarrhea.

Zinc

This is also the stuff used to galvanize steel, but that is for another book. Zinc can be measured, and since about 30 percent of zinc is absorbed in the proximal bowel, some loss can be expected in weight loss patients. Non-specific syndromes of deficiency such as rashes on the face and limbs, hair loss, skin ulcers, poor appetite, lethargy, taste abnormalities, or an assortment of other non-specific syndromes have been attributed to zinc. Taking a vitamin that includes zinc is a good preventative measure.

The Host of Other Minerals

Every month in some magazine they list another mineral or element that is the key to life. Some months it is iodine, copper, selenium, and a host of others. Some vitamins have everything in them, including these trace elements. We know of the toxicity of some of these and not of others, and no doubt there will be an article about Einsteinium, or some other very small element which someone with a lab and a few patients will publish. Again, supplementation of some of these elements is not a problem but some are not needed and some might be harmful. There is an old saying, "just because a couple of aspirin are good doesn't mean you need to take the whole bottle."

Iron Stores

The recommend dose of Ferrous Sulfate or Ferrous Gluconate is 300-350 mg per day. This should not be taken with calcium. Chromagen forte does provide a better source of iron than the other two, but this must be obtained by prescription.

Vitamin Chart

	One A Day	Flintstones	Centrum Chew	Vista
Vitamin A	100%	100%	70%	100%
Vitamin D	100%	100%	100%	100%
Vitamin E	100%	100%	100%	167%
Vitamin K	31%	0%	13%	75%
Thiamin (B1)	100%	100%	100%	800%
Riboflavin (B2)	100%	100%	100%	765%
Niacin (B3)	100%	100%	100%	80%
Pyridoxine (B6)	100%	100%	100%	700%
Folate	100%	100%	100%	100%
Calcium	16%	10%	11%	15%
Iron	100%	100%	100%	22%
Zinc	100%	100%	100%	73%
Vitamin C	200%	100%	100%	200%

Calcium Supplements

Viactive	500 mg Calcium Carbonate 25% Vit. D 50% Vit. K
Cal-100	1000 mg Calcium Carbonate (dissolves in liquid)
Citracal (ultradense)	2 tablets 400 mg Calcium Citrate
Tums	500 mg of Calcium Carbonate
Tums 500	1250 Calcium Carbonate

Calcium and iron should NOT be taken together.

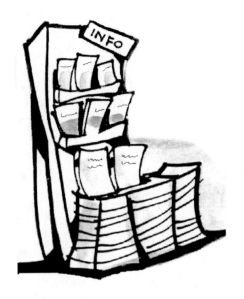

Appendix Four

Resources

Web Sites to Visit

A number of resources are available to patients, family members, and physicians to learn about the various surgeries:

http://www.obesityhelp.com

This is the premier site for weight loss surgery information. It contains data rating hospitals, describing the procedures, and has various forums. Using this site, you can post your before and after photographs. There are physician-moderated chats, plus chats that occur round the clock, plus a quarterly magazine.

http://www.asbs.org

This is the official site for the American Society for Bariatric Surgery. It has a little about the history of the surgery and why the surgery is done, as well as a membership list that is available to you.

http://www.doctorsimpson.com

Okay, so I am throwing in a little shameless self-promotion here. We are proud of our site, as it has information for post-operative diets for patients who have had the duodenal switch, Roux-en-Y, and the lap-band. Our own patients keep the message board going with some levity and humor.

http://groups.yahoo.com/group/WLS_uncensored

This is a free discussion list about almost any weight loss surgery: the good, the bad, and the ugly. A lot of patients post at this site. It is hosted by Sue Widemark, who some weight loss surgeons believe is the devil incarnate. On Sue's forum all sides of the weight loss surgery issue can be debated. Sometimes the debates are intense; sometimes they are a lot of fun.

http://www.duodenalswitch.com

For those contemplating the duodenal switch, this site that will provide you with a list of the physicians who regularly offer it, as well as a lot of other useful information. This site not only has a lot of references for patients, it will also link you to other great sites such as the yahoo forums for the duodenal switch.

http://groups.yahoo.com/group/SmartBandsters

This Yahoo group is dedicated to the adjustable laparoscopic band. They provide you with a number of links, and helpful information. The forum always has a good discussion about the lap-band.

http://www.obesitylaw.com

This is a legal service for morbidly obese people and offers advice in a variety of matters. Walter Lindstrom had RNY surgery after winning a battle with the insurance company. There are a number of useful articles in this site.

http://www.inamed.com

This company has the only approved lap-band in the United States. Their website is a great source of information about the lap-band.

http://www.oregoncenter.com

Probably the best website in the country about the RNY gastric bypass. Dr. Flannigan's site is crisp and informative.

Bibliography

General Articles

Gastrointestinal Surgery For Severe Obesity. Proceedings of a National Institutes of Health Consensus Development Conference. March 25-27, 1991, Bethesda, MD. Am J Clin Nutr, 1992. 55(2 Suppl): p. 487S-619S.

This is the consensus statement that we quoted from earlier in the book.

Robert E. Brolin. *Bariatric Surgery and Long-term Control of Morbid Obesity*. JAMA 2002 288: 2793-2796.

Dr. Brolin has been around a long time and has published a lot in this field.

Ali H. Mokdad; Earl S. Ford; Barbara A. Bowman; William H. Dietz; Frank Vinicor; Virginia S. Bales; James S. Marks *Prevalence of Obesity, Diabetes, and Obesity-Related Health Risk Factors, 2001*. JAMA. 2003;289:76-79.

Kevin R. Fontaine; David T. Redden; Chenxi Wang; Andrew O. Westfall; David B. Allison. *Years of Life Lost Due to Obesity*. JAMA. 2003;289: 187-193.

In spite of what some groups wish you to believe, obesity costs years of your life—see my introduction.

Build And Blood Pressure Study. 1959, Chicago Society of Actuaries.

An old study that shows that you have higher blood pressure when you look like a pear.

Blair, D.F. and L.W. Haines, *Mortality Experience According to Build At Higher Durations*. Society of Actuaries, 1966. **18**: p. 35-46.

M. J. Friedrich. *Epidemic of Obesity Expands Its Spread to Developing Countries*. JAMA 2002 287: 1382-1386.

Stevens, J., et al., *The Effect of Age on the Association Between Body-Mass Index and Mortality* [see comments]. N Engl J Med, 1998. 338(1): p. 1-7.

Hubert, H.B., et al., *Obesity As An Independent Risk Factor In Gross Obesity.* Circulation, 1983. 67: p. 968-977.

Health Implications of Obesity. NIH Consensus Development Conference Statement. Ann Int Med, 1985. 103: p. 1073-77.

Drenick, E.J., et al., *Excessive Mortality And Causes of Death In Morbidly Obese Men.* JAMA, 1980. 243: p. 443-5.

Sjostrom, L., et al., *Swedish Obese Subjects (SOS). Recruitment For An Intervention Study And A Selected Description Of The Obese State.* Int J Obes Relat Metab Disord, 1992. 16(6): p. 465-79.

Sjostrom, C.D., et al., *Reduction In Incidence Of Diabetes, Hypertension And Lipid Disturbances After Intentional Weight Loss Induced By Bariatric Surgery: The Sos Intervention Study.* Obes Res, 1999. 7(5): p. 477-84.

Willett, W.C., et al., Weight, *Weight Change And Coronary Heart Disease In Women. Risk Within The "Normal" Weight Range.* JAMA, 1995. 273: p. 461-5.

Eric Scholosser. *Fast Food Nation. The Dark Side of the All-American Meal.* Harper Collins Publishers.

Diabetes and Obesity

Ali H. Mokdad, Barbara A. Bowman, Earl S. Ford, Frank Vinicor, James S. Marks, and Jeffrey P. Koplan. *The Continuing Epidemics of Obesity and Diabetes in the United States.* JAMA 2001 286: 1195-1200.

Keen, H., *The Incomplete Story Of Obesity And Diabetes*, in *Proceedings of the First International Congress on Obesity*, A. Hayward, Editor. 1975, Newman Publishing Co Ltd: London. p. 116-127.

Report of the United States National Commission on Diabetes to the Congress of the United States, in *Publication Number 76-1021*. 1975, U.S. Department of Heath, Education and Welfare: Bethesda, Maryland.

Beirman, E.L., J.D. Bagdade, and D.J. Porte, *Obesity and Diabetes. The Odd Couple*. Am J Clin Nutr, 1968. **21**: p. 1434-7.

Colditz, G.A., et al., *Weight As A Risk Factor For Clinical Diabetes In Women*. Am J Epidemiol, 1990. **132**: p. 501-13.

Van Itallie, T.B., *Health Implications Of Overweight and Obesity in the United States*. Ann Intern Med, 1985. **103**(6, Pt 2): p. 983-988.

Hartz, A.J., et al., *Relationship Of Obesity To Diabetes: Influences Of Obesity Level And Body Fat Distribution*. Prev Med, 1983. **12**: p. 351-7.

Bennett, O.H., et al., *Epidemiologic Studies Of Diabetes In The Pima Indians*. Rec Prog Horm Res, 1976. **32**: p. 333-6.

Kalkoff, R.K., et al., *Relationship of Body Fat Distribution to Blood Pressure, Carbohydrate Tolerance, and Plasma Lipids In Healthy Obese Women*. J Lab Clin Med, 1974. **102**: p. 621-7.

Surgery for Kids and Adults (old and young)

Jeffrey B. Schwimmer, Tasha M. Burwinkle, and James W. Varni *Health-Related Quality of Life of Severely Obese Children and Adolescents*. JAMA 2003 289: 1813-1819.

Rand, C.S. and A.M. Macgregor, *Adolescents Having Obesity Surgery: A 6-Year Follow-Up*. South Med J, 1994. **87**(12): p. 1208-13.

Breaux, C.W., *Obesity Surgery In Children*. Obes Surg, 1995. **5**(3): p. 279-284.

Strauss, R.S., L.J. Bradley, and R.E. Brolin, *Gastric Bypass Surgery In Adolescents With Morbid Obesity*. J Pediatr, 2001. **138**(4): p. 499-504.

Macgregor, A.M. and C.S. Rand, *Gastric surgery in morbid obesity. Outcome in Patients Aged 55 Years And Older*. Arch Surg, 1993. **128**(10): p. 1153-7.

Murr, M.M., M.R. Siadati, and M.G. Sarr, *Results Of Bariatric Surgery For Morbid Obesity In Patients Older Than 50 Years.* Obes Surg, 1995. **5**(4): p. 399-402.

Dolan, K., Creighton, L., Hopkins, G., Fielding, G. *Laparoscopic Gastric Banding in Morbidly Obese Adolescents.* Obes Surg, 2003. 13(1): p 101-104

Other fun stuff

Samara Joy Nielsen; *Barry M. Popkin Patterns and Trends in Food Portion Sizes*, 1977-1998 JAMA. 2003;289:450-453.

Donald A. Redelmeier and Matthew B. Stanbrook. *Television Viewing and Risk of Obesity.* JAMA 2003 290: 332.

David S. Ludwig. *The Glycemic Index: Physiological Mechanisms Relating to Obesity, Diabetes, and Cardiovascular Disease.* JAMA 2002 287: 2414-2423. A good article, and the book is also an outstanding purchase.

New Glucose Revolution: *The Authoritative Guide to the Glycemic Index— the Dietary Solution for Lifelong Health*. Published by Marlow and Co. Second Edition, by Jennie Brand-Miller, Thomas M.S. Wolever, Kaye Foster-Powell, Stephen Colagiuri

Hess, et al. *Biliopancreatic Diversion with a Duodenal Switch,* Obesity Surgery, 8, 1998; 267-282. **From the pioneer who put this operation together.**

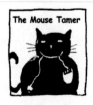

Professional Manuscript Services

by

Yvonne Gray

Book design, graphic arts, editing

www.themousetamer.com